VIBRANT AND CLEAR: *How to Be Acne Free, Naturally!*

by

TONI ANN JOHNSON

To my mother, for all she taught me about skin care.

To Len, for his love and support.

Dear Reader,

Thank you for joining me here. What follows was originally conceived for friends and family who frequently asked how I'd overcome acne to achieve smooth, healthy skin. I began making notes about remedies I'd discovered over the years, then I researched these cures further to corroborate how and why they worked.

Did you know that there are affordable, effective ways to control acne and get great skin without harsh, expensive medications? I didn't, until I'd already spent way too much money and suffered horrible, humiliating side effects, only to find that my skin was still not clear. Many acne medications come with negative side effects ranging from yeast infections, to peeling, raw skin, to potential liver damage. And for all this you pay handsomely. I'm going to share some inexpensive options for managing your acne that may actually benefit your health rather than compromise it.

Please note, however, that I am not a doctor and this information should not be considered medical advice. Results vary from person to person and since I can't know of existing conditions you may have that could make my suggestions inappropriate for you, please be sure to consult your healthcare professional before using any regimen, food, or supplement recommended here.

I hope what you find in these pages helps lead you to the gorgeous, healthy skin you desire.

Warmly and with thanks,
Toni Ann Johnson

CONTENTS

INTRODUCTION

As a young teenager, my skin was creamy-caramel and perfect. People would stop me on the street and ask, "What do you use for skincare?"

I'd shrug thinking, "Skincare? What's *that?*"

At age 13, then 14, I didn't use anything in particular. It was just luck. I washed my face with whatever my mom kept in the bathroom, which was usually Ivory Soap. Occasionally we'd try something different if it happened to be on sale. A cousin of mine was using Noxema Skin Cream at the time and when she visited I'd use that. There were no problems with my skin, so I didn't bother to consider what I *should* be using. Nor did I use moisturizer or sunscreen—it was the 70s and I didn't know the risks of sun exposure, or the benefits of sun protection.

The summer I turned 15 two events adversely affected my skin. Early that summer I went to cheerleading camp. The food was unappealing, so candy bars purchased in the snack shop substituted for most meals. I returned home with twenty-four pimples. I remember the number, because I kept a diary at the time and I'd written it down. My skin looked horrendous—its worst ever, but it cleared up quickly. Once I was home, back to my regular diet, sleep-patterns and twice daily face washings, things were ok.

Later that summer I traveled with my aunt and cousin, the one who used Noxema, to Barbados. For two weeks we baked in the sun sans sunscreen. We did, however, slather on baby oil alloyed with iodine with the hopes of getting deeper tans. I burned at first, but eventually tanned even more deeply than I thought possible. I got so dark that my own mother looked right past me when I arrived at the airport.

"Mom! I'm right here," I said, standing in front of her, my skin toasted to a crisp.

She looked down, leaned back and frowned. "I didn't give birth to any babies as brown as you!"

That fall, as I was entering 10th grade, I noticed my skin was drier than I recalled it being. And there were lines on my face for the first time. They were particularly pronounced on my forehead, an area that had been sunburned. Nearly a decade after that I developed severe, cystic acne in the same area. Though there's no causality that I can be certain of, it *was* uncanny that my most severe breakouts were in the exact same spot that had been sun-damaged. What I *am* certain of is that acne combined with wrinkled, sun-damaged skin is no fun to look at.

After the bad sunburn, years went by and I had little difficulty with my pristine skin. The only flaws were those pesky lines on my forehead. But by age 24, my good skin luck ran out. My mother suffered with oily skin and breakouts, and while I'd thought I'd escaped that bad gene, it caught up with me. Adult acne wreaked havoc, and my face was so filled with pimples and marks, there were days when I was too embarrassed to leave my apartment.

My friend Claudia, an actress in New York City where I lived at the time, recommended a dermatologist who'd helped her. I began seeing Dr. Frederic Fenig, who prescribed an antibiotic called Minocin. He also explained that I needed to stop using oil-based foundation *and* the Vitamin E oil I was putting on my face. (I thought it would heal pimples.) I didn't realize the connection between breakouts and pore-clogging oils. Once I discontinued the Vitamin E, stopped using oil-based foundation, and took the antibiotic, my skin improved. I wasn't completely acne free, but the medication gave me some control. But when I'd stop taking the Minocin the acne would flare up again. Not as bad as it had been, but bad enough that I still needed help.

Eventually, to try to mitigate this, Dr. Fenig prescribed a low dose of Retin A. After some initial adjustment wherein my skin peeled a bit more severely than I was comfortable with, it calmed down and looked pretty spectacular. Retin A also had the added benefit of peeling away old, damaged skin and revealing new, younger looking skin, so the lines on my forehead were minimized and I looked better than I had when I was in high school.

While I remained on both the Minocin and the Retin A, I was smooth and pristine. Unfortunately, my doctor didn't recommend that I *stay* on the Minocin indefinitely and so when I went off it I'd break out again, even while on the Retin A. The breakouts were infrequent and *much* milder than before either medication, but whatever it was that was causing me to breakout was not completely under control. In addition to that, the Minocin caused recurring yeast infections. Not nice.

After being on the low doses of Retin A for some time, its efficacy began to wane and a stronger dose was prescribed. Again, the peeling began and my face was red and unattractive.

Around that time, my health insurance coverage lapsed and I was forced to give up all medications and wing it on my own. My skin, surprisingly, began to calm down. Serendipitously, around that same time, I began working out at the Y, running, using the stationary bike and sitting in the steam room regularly. At the time, I didn't make the connection between the running, the steam and my skin clearing up, but I enjoyed a slight respite from breakouts. It still broke out, occasionally, but less severely than it had previously.

The running caused me to sweat, which helped my body to expel toxins. It also got my blood circulating, which brought nutrients to the skin. The steam helped open the pores, further clearing them out. Also, I was drinking more water, because the exercise made me thirsty. All this proved to be salutary for the acne, but I didn't attribute its improvement to anything I was doing; I thought it had just gone through a phase and was now better.

Then I moved from New York to California and didn't have access to the gym anymore. There was no track available to me, so I was just walking around a neighborhood. This was good exercise, but I didn't sweat much and I did not have a steam room to clear out my pores. My acne returned and slowly got worse.

After a year, my skin was so bad that a friend's young daughter looked my face over one day and asked with concern, "Do you have the chicken pox?"

I realized that I actually looked scary. I began staying in a lot, because I didn't want anyone to see me. Isolating myself due to embarrassment was one of the hardest things about having acne. I felt ugly, and even unlovable. It impeded my life.

At the time, I didn't have the money to see a doctor, but a couple of months went by and when I was able to afford it, I went to a new dermatologist and requested Minocin. He gave me some, but he also prescribed Retin A in a dosage stronger than I'd previously used. I asked him about the lower dosage, but he refused to prescribe that, claiming it wouldn't be effective enough.

The Retin A destroyed my skin! By this time, I was in my early 30s and my skin wasn't as oily as it had been just a few years early. The stronger Retin A dried my skin severely. It peeled in deep groves that bled, and the breakouts continued. He said to give it some time, which I did, but after a couple of months of being embarrassed to be seen in public, I stopped everything, including visiting that doctor.

An aesthetician helped heal the damage from the Retin A, but even bi-monthly facials didn't keep my skin from breaking out.

I went to another dermatologist and implored her to prescribe Accutane. This did the trick. I had not one breakout while on the medication and my skin looked immaculate. But I had to undergo blood tests for potential liver damage. And I had to take birth control pills, because a pregnancy while on this medication would result in alien baby. And to top it off, several months after I'd finished the course of treatment the acne returned!

Eventually, I learned ways to successfully manage my acne without harsh medicines that came with side effects. Much of what I learned not only cleared my acne, but also improved the quality of my skin and enhanced my overall health. This negative experience turned out to be a catalyst that led to positive changes in my appearance and in my life.

If you're suffering from acne and troubled by what it's doing to your looks and self-esteem, and you aren't in a position to see a dermatologist regularly, or you just don't want to take medicine, be encouraged. There *are* ways to control it that are actually inexpensive and good for you. You may have to try a few different things before you find what works, but I'm excited to present what I've learned with you. I'm also confident that once you have all the information you'll be able to incorporate some of these options and be on your way to flawless skin.

FASTING

When you stop eating, it's amazing how the skin clears up. **But don't worry this chapter is *not* about advocating fasting for acne control.** What I want to share is simply what fasting can teach us about digestion and its relationship to acne.

In the early 90s, I did the controversial "Master Cleanse," a fast wherein you drink a combination of pure lemon juice, water, maple syrup and cayenne pepper. While on the fast you also drink a laxative tea at night and a glass of water with salt in it in the morning-- "a salt water flush" that causes elimination. Eventually, you empty your digestive tract completely.

The benefits of this are widely dismissed by doctors. Fasting, in general, is not deemed necessary by the medical community, and is in fact considered potentially harmful. While I still appreciate fasting (briefly) myself, I don't disagree. Friends of mine have, indeed, hurt themselves during fasts. And I understand that the seemingly pervasive advice in the alternative healing community to "detox" *may* be superfluous, because our kidneys and liver are designed to do that for us. However, my *personal* experience with fasting was spectacular. I looked and felt fantastic. That doesn't mean I'm recommending it. Acne can be controlled without it. But because of the wonderful results, I had to conclude that *something* about the fast did my body good.

One thing the Master Cleanse did for me was turn my skin from pimply and bumpy, to smooth as glass in less than two weeks. I glowed.

Research recently led me to an acne forum wherein someone wrote that she'd fasted on nothing but water, and it had completely cleared her acne. Other similar testimonials corroborate that experience. So, while the lemon, cayenne pepper and maple syrup may be a great combination, it's unlikely that any one of them is *essential* for eradicating acne. Water is wonderful for the skin, and I recommend drinking lots of it, but if you're an acne sufferer, you've probably already tried drinking gallons of water, only to find that it, alone, does not eradicate acne. If drinking water was all that was necessary to cure acne, dermatologists would be broke, and so would the companies that make acne medications.

What *does* seem to have an affect on acne is *empty intestines*. I'm still not advocating fasting, but there does seem to be causality between the contents, or lack there of, in the intestines and acne. When the colon (the main part of the large intestine) is empty, acne goes away. Why is that?

The colon is home to copious intestinal flora, including bacteria.

There are two types of bacteria known to contribute to acne: Propionibacterium Acnes and Staphylococcus Aures. Did you know that both can be found on the surface of the skin *and* in the intestines? I did not know this until recently, but it illuminated my own experience with acne and getting rid of it.

The fact that fasting clears acne suggests that these bacteria are reduced when there's no food in the intestines. What can we do with this information? We have to *eat* to live, right? Fasting is certainly *not* an effective way to treat acne long-term, but it does give us clues about the connection between the digestive system and our skin. If it's bacteria in our digestive tract that's contributing to our acne breakouts, what we must figure out is how to control the bacteria as effectively as fasting does. We will want to minimize the "bad" bacteria (which is what antibiotics prescribed for acne do) and encourage the "good" bacteria (which antibiotics don't do). This *battle of the bacteria* is what brings me to the next chapter and the advice I received that finally made a difference...

References:

Fasting and Acne
http://ayur-help.blogspot.com/2011/01/fasting-to-cure-acne-get-clear-skin-in.html
April 25, 2011

http://www.acne.org/messageboard/Fasting-cured-acne-t221108.html
April 25, 2011

Acne Bacteria
http://web.mst.edu/~microbio/BIO221_1998/P_acnes.html
April 25, 2011

http://en.wikipedia.org/wiki/Staphylococcus_aureus

http://www.textbookofbacteriology.net/staph.html

April 25, 2011

ALOE VERA JUICE

One day while lamenting the misery of my adult acne to my friend Denise, she told me about a mutual friend of ours who'd cleared her skin by drinking aloe vera juice and taking acidophilus capsules.

I hadn't heard anything about the effect of aloe vera on acne, but I'd seen jugs of the juice at my local Trader Joe's, and had wondered what its benefits were. Hearing that it could potentially cure acne piqued my interest.

The jug said to drink 2—8 oz. It tasted, in my opinion, *terrible!* But, the directions said you could mix it with other juices without compromising its efficacy, so I tried that.

Sometimes I mixed it with grape juice, other times I used orange juice. I drank about 6 to 8 ounces a day the first week. It seemed to have a very slight laxative effect, but not nearly as harsh as a regular laxative. It didn't upset my stomach or send me running to the toilet. After drinking it for 3 days, I realized I had not had any new acne breakouts. Not *one*. This was unusual for me—I tended to break out daily.

After a week, there were still no new breakouts. I hadn't even tried adding the acidophilus capsules at that point. I was amazed.

This was back in 1999, and I've been drinking aloe vera juice regularly ever since.

What is it about Aloe vera juice that helps control acne?

While working on an earlier book, *VIBRATING YOUTH*, I did some research on aloe vera juice and came across a paper published online that detailed a study proving that the juice reduced bacteria in the colon. This paper is fairly easy to locate via a google search. It's called: "Effect Of Orally Consumed Aloe Vera Juice On Gastrointestinal Function In Normal Humans."

The study showed reduced bowel transit time and reduced bacteria in the stool among the participants who drank small amounts of aloe vera juice three times a day.

As it turns out, aloe vera juice, when ingested, enters the digestive tract and works to minimize the presence of the bacteria that cause acne: Propionibacterium Acnes and Staphylococcus Aureus. *This* is why drinking Aloe Vera juice helps to control acne. As I mentioned in the chapter on fasting, acne-causing bacteria can be found both in the intestines and on the surface of the skin.

I experienced relief from acne when I fasted (completely clearing my colon) *and* when I drank aloe vera juice. In both cases, my digestive tract was being cleansed. The fasting cleared it out, which reduced the bacteria. But the juice killed the bacteria, ("cleaning" it from my colon) without fasting.

I've read articles that posit there's no link to diet and acne, but empirical evidence says there *is.* At least for me there is, and maybe for you, too. Diet doesn't affect *everyone's* acne, because everyone's body doesn't produce the same bacteria in identical amounts.

Your acne may not be the same as mine, or someone else's, but if you do have a proliferation of bacteria in your colon, aloe vera juice will help you.

Hormones largely contribute to acne as well. While this is essentially indisputable, given teenage acne and the fact that women tend to break out more when they menstruate, I know that in my case bacteria is the more nefarious culprit. Once I began drinking aloe vera juice regularly, the breakouts I suffered shortly before and during menstruation were significantly reduced; more often, there were none at all.

So, even though hormones contribute to increased oil production, if the internal and external bacteria are controlled, breakouts from the extra oil (sebum) are not inevitable.

Think of aloe vera juice functioning similarly to the way an antibiotic prescribed for acne works. The antibiotic reduces bacteria and inflammation. Aloe vera juice reduces bacteria and works as an anti-inflammatory as well. But what's better about aloe vera juice is that it doesn't compromise the intestinal flora the way antibiotics do. Antibiotics minimize the "good" bacteria leading to a proliferation of yeast that causes infections in some people. Once you get a yeast infection, it can be difficult to get rid of, and yeast can cause a host of undesirable problems in the body.

If you're suffering from acne I urge you to give aloe vera juice a try. Be sure to buy the "pure" juice, not a brand that adds sugar. The taste, depending on the brand, can be difficult to get used to, to put it mildly. My friend Tracy called the taste, "ghastly." But don't let that scare you. Some brands taste better than others. If you buy the pure aloe vera juice, you can mix it with other juices (preferably unsweetened) and it will still work.

Begin with 4 to 6 oz a day. I recommend using it first thing in the morning and/or after your evening meal. You might want to take it when you take your vitamins, making it part of a regimen. It might irritate your stomach a little at first. Some people have reported that it gives them gas. If so, reduce the amount until you can tolerate at least 4 oz.

If you're still breaking out, work up to 6 to 8oz. Track your breakouts. If after a week of drinking 8oz a day, you're still breaking out as much as you were, then it probably isn't going to work and you shouldn't continue. I noticed a change almost immediately. My advice pertains to people whose bodies respond as mine did.

If it seems to be working for you, you notice a *reduction* in breakouts, but it hasn't completely eradicated it at 8oz, you can work up to drinking more. I no longer have to drink it daily, but when I do, I'll typically drink a 10—12oz. glass, either in the morning or at night, after dinner. The time of day doesn't seem to make a difference, but I find that remembering to do it in the morning and/or evening helps it to become habitual. One of the keys to ensuring its efficacy is being *consistent*. At first, drink it regularly, each day.

Like exercise, you have to make your skin care routines a habit if you want to see results. Once your skin clears, you may be able to reduce your consumption to a few times a week, especially if you make other dietary changes that I'll suggest later in the book. But at first, drink the juice every day.

Externally

The gel from the aloe vera plant is also excellent for clearing acne breakouts and preventing new ones. It has healing and antibacterial properties. You can purchase aloe vera gel from most drug stores. If you do, be sure to purchase the *pure* gel, not the kind with added dyes and chemicals. Fruit of the Earth is a good brand, because it has no dyes or alcohol. You can find it online.

At night, you can apply the pure gel to clean skin. Depending on the ingredients in your daytime moisturizer or other cosmetics, it might not blend well, so it's often easier to use it at night.

If you're adventurous and have access to an actual aloe vera plant, you can extract the pure gel from the plant itself. I highly recommend that you do this! I've had miraculous results with the pure gel extracted directly from the plant.

There are tutorials on youtube that can take you through the process of doing this. It's easier than it sounds.

Break off or cut a portion of the plant (leaf) at least a few inches long. Very thinly slice off the back, flat part—the whole width and length. The gel will be revealed immediately. Take a spoon or knife and scrape it off.

You can store what you don't use in a plastic container in your refrigerator. Use it as you would the store-bought gel—apply to clean skin at night. Or if you're not wearing makeup, apply anytime. It soothes and heals the skin and quickly minimizes redness. The texture is a bit different from the commercial variety, but don't let that scare you. You can apply over your entire face, or just on the areas that are broken out. On healthy skin, it will tone, moisturize, nourish and minimize bacteria and on skin that's broken out it will help to heal and prevent future breakouts.

References:

Benefits of aloe vera juice
http://www.all4naturalhealth.com/medicinal-uses-of-aloe-vera.html

Reduces inflammation, antibacterial
http://www.livestrong.com/article/289491-what-are-the-benefits-of-aloe-vera-for-acne/

http://www.jstor.org/pss/4252402
April 25, 2011

Kills P. Acnes and S. Aures

http://books.google.com/books?id=EovKwdE8Rm
0C&pg=PA85&lpg=PA85&dq=propionibacterium
+acnes+aloe+vera&source=bl&ots=odnl-
O8E0d&sig=RLHdGCWIAcmZVOfD5dS5mfE9r
0A&hl=en&ei=DPy2Td7oG4fbiAK7utgq&sa=X&
oi=book_result&ct=result&resnum=6&sqi=2&ved
=0CDsQ6AEwBQ#v=onepage&q=propionibacteri
um%20acnes%20aloe%20vera&f=false
April 26, 2011

http://staphinfectioninformation.com/drink-aloe-
vera-juice-3875467a
May 20, 2011

PLAIN YOGURT

As I mentioned earlier, the friend who led me to the Aloe Vera juice told me of good results achieved with a combination of aloe vera juice and acidophilus.

Acidophilus is a *good* bacteria, which means it helps mitigate "bad" bacteria. As I've discussed previously, there are bacteria in our digestive tract that contribute to acne and managing them helps control breakouts.

How do we differentiate between "good" bacteria and "bad?"

When you take an antibiotic and develop a yeast infection this is because the medication kills not only the bacteria you're trying to treat, but it also kills the "good" bacteria (acidophilus) that controls Candida Albicans, an un-friendly, single-celled fungus (sometimes referred to as bacteria). Like bacteria, Candida Albicans lives in the gut among the intestinal flora. This fungus creates yeast. Without the presence of acidophilus to control it, the yeast multiplies and proliferates wildly. When it does, it creates problems for us, which is why it's labeled "bad."

Yeast infections can eventually enter the bloodstream. When they do, the yeast becomes systemic and can create many unpleasant symptoms.

This is one good reason to avoid using prescribed antibiotics to treat your acne, especially if you can treat it with something that's actually good for your body and doesn't cause yeast.

The "friendly bacteria" acidophilus is present in good quality, plain (unsweetened) yogurt. It's in *sweetened* yogurt, too, but I recommend unsweetened yogurt for acne control.

The beneficial bacteria in yogurt promote healthy intestines, which leads to good digestion.

Poor digestion has been linked to acne, because when bowel transit time is slow and food is sitting in the system longer than is ideal, bacterial toxicity has an opportunity to build up.

The skin is one of the pathways through which our body releases toxins. As toxins pass through skin, they come in contact with the sebaceous (oil producing) glands and those glands can become inflamed.

When digestion is good, toxins are minimized, resulting in fewer breakouts.

Eating yogurt containing acidophilus helps reduce one of the undesirable bacterium known to contribute to acne: Staphylococcus Aureus. As I've mentioned previously, the *primary* acne causing bacterium is "Propionibacterium Acnes," however Staphylococcus Aureus is *another* bacterium that contributes to skin eruptions.

When Staphylococcus Aureus and other "bad" bacteria are present without good bacteria to mitigate them, they can accumulate and secrete toxins, which end up in the liver.

Excess toxins make the job of the liver more difficult. The liver is supposed to remove toxins. If your body accumulates too many, however, the liver can become overwhelmed. When that happens, the organ is less efficient at eliminating accumulated toxins. Additionally, an overwhelmed liver can't balance hormones effectively. Hormonal imbalance contributes to the over-activity of the sebaceous glands, making them produce too much oil (sebum). This oil comes in contact with bacteria on the skin, and leads to breakouts.

This is why simply treating the skin alone isn't enough for people with severe acne. The skin is only part of the problem. The problem involves digestion, toxin removal, and hormones.

Yogurt is just one of *many* foods that help with digestion and toxin elimination, but yogurt *is* one that specifically helps acne, by controlling Staphylococcus Aureus.

I recommend eating daily portions of 4 to 8 ounces of plain yogurt (without fillers, sweeteners or coloring) as part of a regimen to control acne. If you aren't a fan of plain yogurt, it can take some getting used to. I mix it with cinnamon and a bit of pure vanilla extract. If I'm craving something sweet I'll add some Stevia. If you must use a sweetener try a natural kind like Stevia, or raw honey. Don't use refined white sugar.

While sugar doesn't *cause* acne, it can contribute to it in some people if their liver isn't particularly strong. Elevated blood sugar levels are one of the things that contribute to the hormonal imbalance that I previously touched upon. It's recently been determined that our bodies respond to sugar as a "toxin." And as I explained, toxins overtax the liver. Hormones are secreted to regulate the glucose levels, and if the liver is working harder than is ideal, those hormones then trigger the sebaceous glands to secrete too much oil, leading to breakouts. To be certain you're getting the acne fighting benefits of the acidophilus, avoid sugar.

Externally

It wasn't until I began doing some research for this book that I happened upon articles that recommended using yogurt as a mask on the skin. The acne forums have repeated accounts of people using plain yogurt on their face with excellent results. It is said to reduce the redness and clean the pores. Most of the advice recommends smearing the plain yogurt on the face and leaving it on until it dries and tightens.

You don't need much. A teaspoon should be enough. You can either wipe it over the entire face, or apply small amounts over the areas that are acne prone. I use a cotton ball, dip it in the yogurt, and put in on my entire face as you would other types of skin masks.

Once it's dry, use a warm wet washcloth to rub the dried yogurt off. You may want to follow it with a toner and moisturizer.

When I've tried this myself, my skin seems to love it. As the yogurt dries on my face, it feels like my pores are tightening.

Once I rub it off, it leaves my skin clean, but also soft. The yogurt moisturizes as it reduces surface bacteria, so you're not left with that stripped, dry feeling that conventional acne products can leave you with.

If you drink aloe vera juice and eat plain yogurt regularly, hopefully you won't *need* to do a yogurt mask. But if you're in the early stages of trying to recover from severe acne, I do recommend that you drink the juice, eat plain yogurt, AND consider applying the plain yogurt to your skin.

How Often?

If your acne is mild, you don't need to do the mask more than twice a week. If your acne is severe drink the aloe vera juice (or one of the other options I'll suggest later), eat the plain yogurt, and apply the plain yogurt to your skin daily, let it dry, then remove it with a clean washcloth. You can even sleep with it on and wash off in the morning.

If the idea of smearing yogurt on your face doesn't appeal to you, I'm going to suggest some less messy options later. But given that it's safe, inexpensive, and easy to find, it's worth a try.

References:

Yogurt's benefit to liver
http://www.personal-nutrition-guide.com/detox-food.html

http://www.ncbi.nlm.nih.gov/pubmed/21048484
April 26, 2011

Yogurt mask

http://www.myacnecream.net/yogurt-for-treating-acne
April 26, 2011
http://www.associatedcontent.com/article/634893/yogurt_the_cure_for_serious_acne.html?cat=69
April 26, 2011

Acidophilus kills Staphylococcus Aures
http://www.lactic-acid-bacteria.net/lactobacillus/Lactobacillus-Acidophilus-dual-coated/?sms_ss=twitter&at_xt=4d3fbee74cfef7a2,0

http://www.innvista.com/health/nutrition/biotics/proborg.htm
April 26, 2011

Is Sugar Toxic?
http://www.nytimes.com/2011/04/17/magazine/mag-17Sugar-t.html?pagewanted=all
April 30, 2011

GREEN TEA

Can drinking green tea help control acne? In my experience, yes it can. Green tea is antibacterial and it's high in antioxidants that help reduce acne breakouts. Sometimes when I'm traveling, if I can't find aloe vera juice, I'll drink lots of green tea instead. If I drink enough, it works just as well, because like aloe vera juice, green tea kills bacteria known to cause acne: both Propionibacterium Acnes and Staphylococcus Aureus.

If you try aloe vera juice and find it doesn't work for you, or if it *does* work, but you just don't like it, green tea can be an effective alternative.

Even if you're happy with the aloe vera juice, once your acne is beginning to come under control with the juice and the yogurt, it can be beneficial to substitute a few days a week with green tea *instead* of aloe vera juice.

It hasn't been my experience, but I've read that some people can develop a dependency on aloe vera juice to help them move their bowels. If you mix up the days, drinking aloe vera juice a few times a week, and green tea a few times—you might try switching them every other day—you won't run into the problem of becoming dependent on the juice to go to the bathroom.

On your "TEA" days, I recommend drinking at least two 8—10 oz cups a day to help control acne. For me, it works best to drink the tea in the morning, because it contains caffeine and can disrupt your sleep if you have it late in the day. (Be sure to brush your teeth after drinking it, because it can stain them.) Try decaffeinated green tea if you prefer to have it in the evening. When you're healing from acne, you definitely don't want to lose sleep, because your skin heals best when you're sleeping.

Another wonder of green tea in the treatment of acne is that it's also said to help regulate hormones. This helps combat acne as well, because, as I've mentioned, hormonal imbalance can lead to the overproduction of sebum, which, when combined with bacteria, causes pimples. So, drink up!

Externally

Scouring acne forums while doing research for this book, I also found that people get relief from acne by putting green tea on their skin, using it as a toner. Upon further research I found that this is actually recommended by skin experts.

Try it in the morning. After you drink your tea, squeeze some of the excess liquid in the tea bag onto a cotton ball, or dip the ball in what's left of the tea. After washing and drying, go over your entire face with the tea soaked cotton and let it dry.

It has the same antibacterial effect *on* the skin that it has internally, attacking both Propionibacterium Acnes and Staphylococcus Aureus (which are present in the intestines as well as on the surface of the skin). It is said to be as effective at combating these bacteria (on the skin) as Benzyol Peroxide. In my opinion, it's *better*, because green tea also has anti-aging benefits.

After you've applied the green tea to your face or other acne prone areas, you can apply your moisturizer and sunscreen without washing off the tea. Green tea is also said to help protect the skin from the sun. I wouldn't use it as a replacement for sunscreen, but used on the skin regularly, it may help prevent sun damage.

When I use it on my face, I find that it has an astringent effect, minimizing the pores without depleting the skin of moisture. And due to its antibacterial properties, green tea not only begins to clear the skin of existing pimples, regular use will help prevent future breakouts as well.

References:

Effect of Green Tea on P. Acnes and S. Aures
http://www.ncbi.nlm.nih.gov/pubmed/19107860

http://www.naturalacneremedy.com/btf/green-tea-and-acne.html
April 26, 2011

Benefits of Green Tea

http://www.naturalacneremedy.com/btf/green-tea-and-acne.html

Hormones and green tea
http://www.ehow.com/way_5317123_foods-hormone-imbalance.html

http://www.adoctorsguideto.com/topics/hormone-balance/
April 26, 201

APPLE CIDER VINEGAR

For years, I've been drinking "vinegar tea" made with a cup of hot water, two tablespoons of organic (unfiltered) apple cider vinegar, and honey. Like aloe vera juice and green tea, apple cider vinegar works in the digestive system to reduce bacteria, which helps to control breakouts.

You can try apple cider vinegar in place of aloe vera juice and green tea, or you can rotate all three, which is what I often do. Because our bodies don't respond exactly alike, I encourage you to experiment with each of them. All three have benefits and each will help reduce acne-causing bacteria, but one may prove more effective for you than others. Even though I've found aloe vera juice to work best for me, I still love organic apple cider vinegar and use it regularly.

In addition to its help with acne, there are myriad health benefits. Taking apple cider vinegar will aid digestion and help alleviate constipation, which, in turn, will assist the body in eliminating toxins, thus helping to combat acne. Doctors have dismissed *some* of the purported benefits of apple cider vinegar, but acknowledged the truth in others. One of the benefits doctors agree with is that the acetic acid found in apple cider vinegar can help reduce blood sugar.

As you know by now, having read previous chapters, when you're trying to control acne some reports suggest that it's helpful to avoid raising the blood sugar rapidly, because a spike in blood sugar can contribute to breakouts by over-taxing the liver, which leads to excess hormones in the blood (because the liver is too overwhelmed to clear them) and these hormones stimulate sebum production. The extra sebum contributes to breakouts. So, the effect of apple cider vinegar in lowering blood sugar *and* aiding the liver, contributes to clearer skin.

Apple cider vinegar kills *some* (not all) types of bacteria, but I haven't been able to find confirmation that it kills acne-causing bacteria, specifically. It certainly seems to, but unlike aloe vera juice and green tea, I've been unable to locate studies that prove apple cider vinegar kills P. acnes and S. Aures. And yet I do see a benefit when I use it internally and externally. I've also read many testimonials and watched videos that boast excellent acne control results using apple cider vinegar.

The vinegar and water tastes much better with honey, but if you can tolerate it without honey, even better, in my opinion. If you do use the sweetener, I recommend *raw* honey rather than pasteurized, because raw honey has a lower glycemic index and won't spike the blood sugar level as quickly as regular honey, or sugar.

I've read articles suggesting that too much vinegar can cause low potassium levels, and low bone density, so I recommend that you drink one cup at a time, rather than loading up on several cups in one sitting. Also, do consider alternating drinking the vinegar tonic with the aloe vera juice and the green tea. That way, you won't consume the vinegar daily over long periods of time. Try to limit it to no more than four times per week, unless recommended by a doctor or naturopath.

Externally

Apple cider vinegar is an excellent toner for oily, acne prone skin. It can help heal your acne lesions and prevent new ones from forming because apple cider vinegar is similar, chemically, to glycolic acid (also known as "hydroxy**acetic**" acid), which is used by dermatologists in the treatment of acne. The major ingredient in apple cider vinegar is acetic acid so we can see from the similarity to the word "hydroxyacetic" the relationship between acetic acid and glycolic acid. Though they are not identical, the fact that they are very close is what makes apple cider vinegar effective for acne control. Like glycolic acid, acetic acid functions as an exfoliant, sloughing away dead skin cells.

How do you use it?

Mix the vinegar with equal parts water and apply with a cotton ball. You can put the mixture all over the face and use a moisturizer on top of it.

For individual pimples, you can dab a small amount of straight vinegar right on them, and leave it.

I don't recommend putting undiluted vinegar all over your face and leaving it for long periods of time, though, because it can burn your skin. It is, after all, acid. But using straight apple cider vinegar over the entire face for *short* periods of time can be a benefit.

According to dermatologist and author of *Six Weeks to Sensational Skin,* Dr. Loretta Ciraldo, if you test apple cider vinegar on your individual pimples and have no adverse reaction, and rather, find it helps your acne, you *can* use straight apple vinegar; Wipe it over the face, or other acne prone areas and leave it for up to 10 minutes, then wash it off. Dr. Ciraldo claims this can help your acne and prevent future breakouts. Here's a link to her youtube tutorial:

http://www.youtube.com/watch?v=upk3hnnEKxE

Once, not knowing what I was doing, I held a cotton ball with straight vinegar on a large cystic lesion for about 40 to 50 minutes while watching television. I burned my skin and was left with a dark mark that took more than a year to fade.

Never *press* straight vinegar on your skin and leave it there. A dab on a spot means just that—a little dab— uncovered.

Diluting it is the safest way to use it. What's worked best for me is making a toner out of 50% apple cider vinegar and 50% water, wiping over the face and allowing it to dry. Then I put a non-comedogenic moisturizer (usually virgin coconut oil—more on that later) on top of that.

If you're drinking the aloe juice, green tea, or apple cider vinegar, hopefully your breakouts will be under control and you won't need to use this. But until then, the vinegar can be very useful as a toner and to control oil. I don't use it everyday, but if my pores seem enlarged, or if I get blackheads, I find that it works well to clean and minimize them.

Test it and see how your skin reacts. If you find that your skin becomes excessively dry after using it, it may not be appropriate for you. Either discontinue, or try cutting back on how often you apply it. If it burns, your skin may be too sensitive for it, or you may need to further dilute it. If you get good results and decide to incorporate it into your skin care routine, you might consider alternating the use of apple cider vinegar as a toner, with green tea, so that you can get the benefits of both.

References:

Benefits of Apple Cider Vinegar—Acetic Acid
http://www.webmd.com/diet/apple-cider-vinegar

Glycolic Acid
http://www.kaviskin.com/info/glycolicacid.html

April 26, 2011

Apple cider vinegar benefit and similarity to glycolic acid
http://www.youtube.com/watch?v=upk3hnnEKxE
April 26, 2011

AVC benefits acne:
http://www.youtube.com/watch?v=upk3hnnEKxE
May 26, 2011

WHITE TEA

I had never heard of white tea until I began researching this book. While reading up on the acne fighting benefits of *green* tea, I kept seeing information on white tea.

Several sources say that white tea is less processed than green tea. According to what I've read, it's made from the buds and younger leaves of the tea plant that are dried naturally in the sun. It comes from the same plant as green tea, however the process of making green tea doesn't include the buds, only the leaves, and the leaves for green tea are harvested later than they are when making white tea.

White tea also has less caffeine (15mg) than the same sized serving of green tea, which has 20mg. Coffee has an average of about 85mg a cup.

Proponents of white tea claim that it has more "catechins" than green tea. According to The Free Dictionary on line, catechins are defined as: *"phytochemical compounds found principally in green tea. Smaller amounts are contained in grapes, black tea, chocolate, and wine. Considered potent antioxidants."* These antioxidants in white tea are said to fight cancer, diabetes and clogged arteries.

What's consistent with all the articles I've been reading about white tea, is that drinking it promotes healthy skin. Evidence suggests that it's anti-bacterial and anti-fungal. There have been studies that show it is effective in killing the Staphylococcus Aures bacterium, one of the bacterium that can contribute to acne.

There's plenty of anecdotal testimony about white tea from acne sufferers on the message boards. It's inconsistent, though. Some say it helped their acne and some say it didn't. Because the use of white tea is more recent in the US than the use of green tea, it may take a while for scientific evidence confirming its efficacy as an acne treatment to be as pervasive as it is for green tea. And the evidence may ultimately *not* show that it's particularly effective.

I decided to try it, based on the information that it has more antioxidants and less caffeine than green tea. What I noticed immediately is that the taste is milder than that of green tea. I prefer the lighter taste and find that it's pleasant to drink, even without adding any sweetener.

While I like it, for now I can't recommend it for acne with the same confidence I can recommend aloe vera juice, apple cider vinegar and green tea, only because there's less information available at this time. I did want you to know about it, however, so you can research it for yourself, and decide if it's something you want to try. The evidence is strong for white tea's overall benefit to good health, so it can't hurt.

References:

Anti-viril, anti-fungal benefits of white tea (2004 study referenced)
http://www.onewhitetea.com/one_white_tea_facts_benefits.php
April 27, 2011

Caffeine
http://coffeetea.about.com/od/typesoftea/a/whitetea.htm
April 27, 2011

About White tea
http://teaguardian.com/nature_of_tea/whites.html
April 27, 2011

WATER

One winter, before I learned about fasting, or aloe vera juice, I was acting in a play at the Cleveland Playhouse. During rehearsals, which ran several hours each day, we sat at a long table (large cast). Upon the table were pitchers of water and small paper cups. For a few weeks, I was drinking a paper cupful (about 3 oz.) at least twice each hour.

At the end of week two, I noticed that my skin was clearer than usual. There was nothing different about my routine except for drinking water twice per hour for several hours a day. I assumed that was the reason my skin cleared up, however, I can't find any research to back this up. And when I tried using water, years later, to clear my skin when it was particularly broken out, the effort failed.

One of the things skin experts consistently say is that drinking plenty of water contributes to good skin. Dermatologists as well as aestheticians have told me that, and I believe them. Until that point, however, I had not thought to drink water twice per hour. Just a few ounces – about 4 oz. every thirty minutes worked wonders for me.

I must admit this is *not* the way I continued drinking water once the rehearsal period was over. The benefits of that water schedule were lost once I resumed my regular routine. I continued to drink water, but not twice per hour, and my acne slowly returned.

It's a bit inconvenient to drink twice per hour for a few reasons, but if you can do it, good for you. Your skin will probably love it. Unfortunately, there's no guarantee it will clear your acne. But perhaps the double dose of water every hour has some positive effect on digestion in *some* people. Water aids elimination. Without enough, stools become too hard, and move through intestines too slowly, resulting in constipation. When digestion is sluggish, and waste is sitting in your body longer than is ideal, toxins are slower to be eliminated and this can contribute to acne.

While drinking a lot of water will help your skin look firmer and more vibrant, because it's hydrated, it's unlikely to cure *severe* acne. People who experience minor, or occasional breakouts may, indeed, find that the extra water is all they need to stay clear.

For me, there have been periods wherein I suffered from very bad acne, and though I drank up to 64oz. of water a day, the breakouts continued. Admittedly, my diet was poor then. I hadn't yet learned what to eat to keep my system running properly, and because I was ingesting a lot of sugar, processed foods, and refined starches, I may have been overtaxing my liver, preventing it from keeping my hormones balanced. Would the water have been more effective had my diet been better? Maybe.

I DO recommend that you drink *plenty* of water. Try to get up to 8 glasses a day, which is the recommendation you've probably heard many times before. Though water alone won't get rid of acne it will *help,* because it will assist your digestive system, improve blood flow, and keep you hydrated. In addition to making you look better, staying hydrated is a benefit to your overall health.

References:

Skin benefits of drinking water
http://www.uwhealth.org/madison-plastic-surgery/the-benefits-of-drinking-water-for-your-skin/26334
April 26, 2011

Water and acne
http://www.naturalacneremedy.com/btf/treat-acne-water.html
April 26, 2011

COCONUT OIL

As I write this, it's been about five years since Anna
Marie Carter, an environmentalist in South Los
Angeles, introduced me to the benefits of food-grade
coconut oil. She made me a meal cooked in virgin
coconut oil, then sent me home with a small jar of it.
It changed my skin and my life.

I began cooking with it, and using it on my skin. At
first, I didn't want to try it on my face, but used it on
my body in place of lotion, and found that my skin
drank up the oil and loved it. It occurred to me that
what we put on our skin is absorbed into our bodies,
and eventually into our bloodstream; so if I wouldn't
eat something, I probably shouldn't put it on my skin
day after day, either. Virgin coconut oil, which
contains no added chemicals, became a staple for
moisturizing my skin.

I read a book called *The Coconut Oil Miracle,* by Bruce Fife, and began learning more and more about how this amazing oil benefits our bodies inside and out. The idea that coconut oil could help with acne contradicted what I understood about oils at the time. Back in my 20s, I'd had a terrible experience putting vitamin E oil on my face, hoping to heal my pimples. It clogged my pores and made my acne worse. But Fife explained that coconut oil is antibacterial and even acts as an exfoliant, helping to remove dead, surface skin cells. He said it would not clog the pores and that used over time, it would clear acne and even fade the marks left by old blemishes.

Still hesitant, I tried it, but only on my forehead. I put on a thin layer before going to bed. The next morning it hadn't caused my skin to break out. In fact, it had helped minimize the inflammation of a small blemish.

Slowly, I began using it on my entire face and found that it actually seemed to control my oily skin. Counter-intuitive, but it was true. When I used the coconut oil at night, I'd wake up with supple skin, but it was not greasy even on my nose, where my pores were generally oiliest. It seemed that when I put things on my skin designed to dry it out, like benzyol peroxide, the skin produced *more* oil than it did when I moisturized with the coconut oil. My skin, when too dry, was compensating by producing more sebum to moisturize itself. When I used the coconut oil, my skin's own rate of sebum production calmed down.

Sometimes when I've mentioned using coconut oil for acne to others, they've told me that it broke their skin out. But with further inquiry, I found out they were using the kind you buy in the drug store. That is *not* what I'm recommending. I'm talking about food-grade, extra virgin coconut oil that you can also eat and cook with. You can get it at Whole Foods, or less expensively, online. As I always say, everyone is different; one person's skin doesn't respond exactly like another's, so, it's possible that extra virgin coconut oil may not benefit your acne, but it should. Coconut oil contains lauric acid, which studies have shown kills the acne causing bacterium, Propionibacterium Acnes.

Internally

For the best results, I recommend including some extra virgin coconut oil in your diet as well as using it topically. As with aloe vera juice, green tea and apple cider vinegar, coconut oil will help control acne causing bacteria (both S. Aures and P. Acnes) in your digestive tract and on your skin.

If you're older than 35 and still dealing with acne, you may be suffering the frustrating reality of having wrinkles *and* pimples. Coconut oil will be a miracle for you, then. If you include it in your diet (at least a tablespoon per day) *and* use it on your skin, in several weeks you'll be amazed by how vibrant and healthy your skin will look.

Don't eat too much. In his book, Fife recommends up to four tablespoons per day, but when I ate that much, I gained weight, despite claims that it aids weight loss. You can benefit from adding as little as one to two tablespoonfuls, (Fife confirms this) and that amount can be achieved without weight gain by simply using it in place of other oils in cooking. Pure, creamy coconut oil actually tastes good enough to use in place of butter on your vegetables. Try it on a baked sweet potato or piece of whole-grain toast. Coconut oil has been previously frowned upon because it's a saturated fat and was thought to clog arteries, but the study that gave it its bad reputation was not done with virgin coconut oil, which doesn't adversely affect cholesterol.

References:

Lauric acid kills Propionibacterium Acnes
http://www.ncbi.nlm.nih.gov/pubmed/19665786
May 7, 2011

Virgin coconut oil has antimicrobial effect on Staphylococcus Aures
http://www.medscape.com/viewarticle/586673_5
May 7, 2011

Coconut oil as an acne cure
http://www.tiana-coconut.com/coconut_oil_acne.html
May 17, 2011

Fife, Bruce. <u>The Coconut Oil Miracle</u>., Penguin: New York, 2004.

Coconut oil and saturated fat
http://www.nytimes.com/2011/03/02/dining/02App e.html?_r=1
June 1, 2011

NEEM OIL

What *is* neem oil? You may not have heard of it. I
hadn't, until my friend Apinya, who owns and runs
RaKsa, a day spa in Culver City, California told me
about it and gave me some as a gift. It comes from the
Neem Tree, found in India, and is made by pressing
the fruit and seeds from the tree.

Natural neem oil has a pungent odor that some may
find intolerable. To me it smells garlicky, but I've
heard the odor described as combination of garlic and
peanuts. You can find neem oil alloyed with other
oils, however, and the strong scent can be
ameliorated. I don't mind the odor so much, but I
would only use it when I'm going to be home, usually
at night. It's not something I'd want to subject others
to. But I love it! It works for acne and other skin
problems.

Unlike coconut oil, which I recommended earlier,
neem isn't something you ingest. In fact, if you
happen to taste it you'll probably regret it. But it's
wonderful for healing acne lesions.

I recommend dipping a cotton swab into the oil and
dabbing it on individual pimples. It reduces the
redness and heals them quickly. I also use it on
mosquito bites, or if I happen to get a scratch. It
works just as well as antibacterial ointment in
preventing infection.

Neem oil is antibacterial, anti-viral, anti-fungal, and anti-inflammatory, and has been shown to reduce the presence of acne-causing Propionibacterium Acnes.

Neem is frequently used in Ayurvedic medicine. Ayurvedic healing, which has its roots in India, tends to involve mental, social, and spiritual wellbeing, in addition to physical wellbeing. Ayurvedics appreciate neem oil's blood purification properties and use it to treat a variety of skin ailments.

If you've never tried one with good results, it may sound risky to use any type of oil on oily skin. But like coconut oil, neem oil kills bacteria and doesn't clog pores. Before you use it all over your face, however, test it on one small area and see what the results are. If it seems to reduce the redness and begin to heal your pimples, then it's likely fine for you to use.

For people with dry or mature skin, I recommend neem oil, in place of more drying types of pimple remedies, like benzyol peroxide. Sometimes with mature skin, when you treat an individual pimple with harsh medications, it can dry out the area beyond the pimple as well. Neem will heal the pimple without depleting the surrounding area of moisture.

References:

Neem oil and propionibacterium acnes

http://books.google.com/books?id=j5PdVtMgVLY
C&pg=PA94&lpg=PA94&dq=neem+oil+propioni
+acnes&source=bl&ots=rIa7WyxLpd&sig=4pNL
TqiPRiD4YS80QoqH1UjCQLM&hl=en&ei=E561
TfzRI8bXiAK54MyvBg&sa=X&oi=book_result&
ct=result&resnum=1&ved=0CBkQ6AEwAA#v=o
nepage&q&f=false
April 28, 2011

Ayurvedics and Neem

http://www.neem-products.com/neem-
ayurveda.html
May 4, 2011

http://neemoilbenefits.org/
May 4, 2011

TEA TREE OIL

I used to use a Tea Tree Oil blemish stick, a gel-based product from The Body Shop, that you dipped an applicator into then dapped onto individual spots. I loved it, and thought it worked well. My skin was *so* bad, however, that it didn't make sense to continue treating each blemish individually. I needed to work on the root cause of the acne. That said, I do recommend tea tree oil for mild acne sufferers.

Some people may not like neem oil (which I recommended previously), because of its pungent odor. Tea tree oil is an essential oil derived from the leaves an Australian plant called Melaleuca Alternifolia, and its scent is fairly pleasant, slightly medicinal, minty, with a hint of pine.

It's proven to be effective in treating acne lesions and has been shown to kill Propionibacterium Acnes and Staphylococcus Aures. It's also antifungal and anti-inflammatory.

One study compared tea tree oil's effects to benzoyl peroxide. They found that while the tea tree oil took a bit longer to work, the results were comparable, and there were fewer side effects.

Tea tree oil can be purchased undiluted, but it's recommended that a 5% solution be used to treat acne lesions. Using straight tea tree oil can cause irritation. Because it might be difficult for individuals to measure 5%, I recommend using a preparation made specifically for acne. The one by The Body Shop is great, as is the one by Burt's Bees. You can find them online.

References:

Does Tea Tree Oil Work?
http://well.blogs.nytimes.com/2011/01/27/remedies
-tea-tree-oil-for-acne/
May 27, 2011

About Tea Tree Oil
http://altmedicine.about.com/od/teatreeoil/a/teatre
eoilacne.htm
May 27, 2011

Tea tree oil and Propionibacterium Acnes and Staphylococcus Aures
http://www.ncbi.nlm.nih.gov/pubmed/7576514
May 27, 2011

CASTOR OIL

My first experience with castor oil was during a bout with "frozen shoulder," a painful, inflammatory joint condition. I was researching anything and everything I could find for relief and stumbled upon castor oil, which has anti-inflammatory properties. Once I got it, I was curious about what else it was used for and I saw that it is sometimes used for acne.

Being acne prone myself, I was skeptical, because it's thick and heavy, unlike coconut oil, which is lighter and absorbs into the skin more quickly. But I kept reading about it, and my fears were somewhat allayed when every article I found claimed that it's non-comedogenic for most people.

Why? A heavy oil that's non-comedogenic? Doesn't sound logical, does it? Castor oil is derived from the Castor Bean and it contains something called Ricinoleic Acid, which gives it anti-bacterial and anti-inflammatory properties. It also contains Undecylenic acid, which is anti-viral and anti-fungal. The combination causes the oil to heal and protect the skin, rather than clog and inflame it, like oils without anti-bacterial and anti-inflammatory properties.

The thing I like about castor oil for *adult* acne, specifically, is how moisturizing and emollient it is. It minimizes lines and wrinkles, while it also works on breakouts, reducing the inflammation and preventing new ones. Having wrinkles and pimples at the same time is a difficult conundrum, because of course you want to minimize the extra oil in your skin, but when you do that, you dry it out, making lines and wrinkles worse. Like coconut oil, castor oil controls acne without drying the skin, but it's thicker than coconut oil and remains on the surface of the skin longer. Despite this, it's actually killing bacteria while it's resting on the skin. It lubricates it, and at the same time, reduces inflammation and minimizes redness.

I probably wouldn't recommend castor oil to treat teenage acne, because extra heavy moisturizing isn't necessary for younger acne-prone skin—it produces enough oil on its own. But if you have adult acne and also lines and wrinkles, castor oil's extra emollience may be great for you.

One added benefit is that castor oil also works as a pain reliever. It's Ricinoleic acid, in addition to giving it its anti-bacterial and anti-inflammatory properties, also makes it an excellent analgesic (pain reducer). If you've ever suffered from severe acne cysts, you're aware that they can be quite painful. You may find relief with castor oil.

When my skin seems extra dry, but it's also breaking out, I use castor oil, applying small amounts to cleansed skin before bed. You can dab it on with a cotton ball, or use your fingers. I generally pat the excess off with a paper towel. Sometimes I'll use it to cleanse my face. When I do this, I begin by applying the oil and massaging my skin with it. Then I take a hot washcloth and hold it over my face for a minute or two. After that, I wipe the oil off with a hot washcloth. What I've found is that the combination of the oil and the steam from the hot cloth, actually helps to unplug the pores. Sounds counter intuitive, but this has been my experience. The first time I did it, I noticed that after I removed the hot cloth, some of the blackheads on my nose began lifting out on their own.

If you decide to give castor oil a try, before using it all over your face, test it on a small portion of your skin, perhaps the chin, overnight, and see how it does. Some people may be allergic to it, so do test it out first.

References:

Castor oil for acne
http://www.ehow.com/how_5047644_treat-acne-castor-oil.html

http://skinverse.com/castor-oils-many-uses-for-beautiful-skin-and-hair.html

Benefits of Castor Oil

June 4, 2011

BAKING SODA

Baking soda, also known as sodium bicarbonate, is chemical salt. This white powder, with its crystalline grains, is great for cleansing the skin. It's a mild abrasive, kills bacteria, and will gently exfoliate without irritating.

To use it, pour about a tablespoon of baking soda into your hand and add just enough water, about a teaspoon or so, to mix it into a paste. Then apply the paste to your face and neck and gently rub in a circular motion all around to cleanse and exfoliate, before rinsing it off completely. It's excellent for oily and acne prone skin, due to its antibacterial properties.

Some acne sufferers, especially teens, may suffer from Keratosis Pilaris, which isn't acne, but is a related condition that occurs when the body produces excess protein in the skin. The protein, called Keratin, builds up, trapping the hair follicle, and eventually it plugs the pore, creating a red bump that looks like a pimple. Exfoliating with baking soda can help alleviate this condition.

As a Mask:

If you like, you can leave the mixture on as a mask. Spread over the face and leave it for 10 to 15 minutes, allowing it to dry. Then take a wet washcloth, wipe off and rinse. Your skin will be clean, but not too dry. It will help clean out the pores and minimize inflammation from pimples.

For Breakouts:
To treat a pimple directly, make a small amount of paste by adding just enough water to a bit of the baking soda and put directly on the spot, allowing it to dry. The baking soda will help draw out the infection, assisting with the healing process.

References:

Baking soda for acne
http://www.bakingsodaacne.com/
May 11, 2011

Antibacterial activity of baking soda
http://www.ncbi.nlm.nih.gov/pubmed/11524862

http://mizar5.com/keyes.html
June 1, 2011

Keratosis Pilaris
http://www.medicinenet.com/keratosis_pilaris/article.htm

June 1, 2011

IODINE

While you're trying to eradicate acne, you may find it helpful to reduce your intake of iodine.

The first dermatologist I saw for my skin over 20 years ago. Dr. Fenig, in New York City, told me that iodine could aggravate my acne. Iodine is a mineral that goes into the bloodstream and if there's more in the blood than the body needs, the excess gets excreted through the sebaceous glands, irritating the pores as it passes through them. The body needs *some* iodine, but too much can cause problems for acne prone people.

Here's a list of some foods that are *very* high in iodine: Kelp, beef liver, turkey, iodized salt and asparagus.

You shouldn't omit iodine entirely. It's easy to get an adequate amount in a balanced diet that includes meats, or fish, some dairy products, and vegetables. Reducing your intake of especially high iodine foods, however, may lead to fewer breakouts.

Iodine and acne
http://www.ehow.com/about_5368460_foods-high-iodine-avoid-acne.html

Foods high in iodine
http://www.mothernature.com/l/The-Doctors-Book-of-Home-Remedies/Acne_2573.html

CHOCOLATE AND SOY

This may be controversial, because the idea that chocolate causes acne has long been debunked. And no scientific evidence has been found linking acne to soy. And yet, both break my skin out. When I still ate sugar, which I now avoid, I was able to eat boatloads of *dark* chocolate containing no milk fat without breaking out. As soon as I ate a small piece of *milk* chocolate, a crowd of zits would invade my face. The same thing happens when I eat soy products, either tofu or soy milk; I break out within a day.

If milk chocolate and soy do not cause acne, then I guess I'm simply allergic to them.

I didn't realize the soy—acne connection until I began doing research for this book. I came across a lot of acne forum chatter that mentioned soy and breaking out. I also found conflicting information that said that soy, because it contains plant estrogens, could be helpful to acne. When I began thinking back to my worst acne bouts, it was during periods wherein I was eating tons of soy. More recently, I conducted my own experiment, drinking some soymilk while visiting a family member. Pimples erupted the next day. Unfortunately I can't explain *why* soy does this to me. But apparently, a lot of people have the same issue with both soy and milk chocolate.

Doctors continually say that there's no link between diet and acne, but if you're an acne sufferer you know your own body; just listen to it and adjust accordingly.

References:

Soy and acne
http://www.quickacneremedy.com/acne-articles/soy-and-acne.html
April 27, 2010

Milk and acne
http://dermatology.cdlib.org/124/original/acne/danby.html
June 4, 2011

REFINED SUGAR AND WHITE FLOUR

Sugar and starches like white flour and white rice can aggravate acne in some people. This is because these foods cause a spike in blood sugar. When blood sugar surges, the pancreas secretes too much insulin. Excess insulin can cause elevated levels of testosterone to enter the blood. (Testosterone, the male sex hormone, can be found in both men and women.) Too much testosterone triggers the sebaceous glands to produce excess sebum (oil), causing clogged pores, which creates a favorable environment for acne bacteria to thrive.

When the hormones are out of balance like this, the liver has to work harder to level them. The liver is tasked with removing toxins from the blood, but it also has to clear excess hormones from the blood. But if the liver is already overworked, trying to clear the blood of toxins, excess hormones can overwhelm it, and so it may not effectively remove them. The hormones then remain in your blood and as mentioned above, cause the body to produce too much sebum, which contributes to acne.

You can help the liver by not overwhelming it with too many toxins. Recently there has been mounting evidence to suggest that sugar, itself, is a toxin. Both sugar and high fructose corn syrup are metabolized by the liver and can overtax it.

According to a study at The University of Colorado, refined sugars and grains may be one of the causes of teenage acne. The study found that unlike the pervasive presence of acne among 18 year olds in modern society, the condition is essentially non-existent in the subsistence society of the Kitava Islanders in Papa New Guinea. Staples of the Kitava Islander diet include: root vegetables, fish, fruit, coconut meat, and coconut oil. They smoke cigarettes, but eat no refined sugars, or refined grains, and they drink no alcohol. Not only is the population free of acne, heart disease and obesity are extremely rare among them, despite the high saturated fat (coconut oil) diet they consume.

The University of Colorado study's findings also corroborated the fact that eating refined sugars and grains led to an overproduction of insulin, resulting in an overproduction of testosterone, which leads to overproduction of sebum. In addition to that, they found that eating refined grains also contributed to keratosis pilaris, a condition common among teens, in which skin cells build up without shedding, blocking the hair follicle and eventually clogging pores.

When my own acne was at its worst, my diet included a hefty amount of sugar and white flour. Over the years, I've cut out refined sugar and white flour as much as possible. This not only helps with acne, but also with weight loss. And it slows the aging process.

While working on my first book, *Vibrating Youth* I discovered that sugar ages you, through a process called "glycation." That was enough to get me to work toward cutting it out. Glycation is a process wherein the sugar in your blood attaches to proteins and forms harmful new molecules called AGE's--"advanced glycation end products." The more sugar you eat, the more of these advanced glycation end products you develop, and they create wrinkles. So if less acne isn't reason enough to avoid sugar, perhaps avoiding wrinkles is. In place of refined sugar, try using Stevia, pure maple syrup, or raw honey. Better still, cut sweeteners out completely, or at least as much as possible.

Refined grains are converted into sugars when ingested; this is why they're part of this discussion and why it's best to minimize them in your diet. Refined grains include: white bread, pasta, white rice, cakes, cookies and sugary cereals. If you're suffering from acne, try eliminating them from your diet for several weeks to see how it affects your skin. In place of refined grains you might try: brown rice, oatmeal, or quinoa. I also like to substitute sweet potatoes in place of refined grains.

Reducing your sugar and refined grain intake *may* help your acne, so it's worth thinking about if you're currently eating white bread and sugar and your skin is breaking out. At the least, making the change will improve your diet, which in turn, will help you age more gracefully and enhance your health.

References:

Sugar and acne
http://worldvillage.com/acne

http://ezinearticles.com/?Acne-and-Diet---Insulin,-Insulin-Resistance,-and-Hormones&id=243622

High glycemic index and acne
http://www.lifescript.com/Health/Conditions/Skin/Battling_Grown-Up_Breakouts.aspx
May 17, 2011

Low glycemic diet and acne
http://www.quickacneremedy.com/acne-articles/Low-Glycemic-Diet-Prevents-Acne.html
May 23, 2011

Teenage acne, diet to blame
http://www.foodnavigator.com/Science-Nutrition/Acne-modern-diet-to-blame
May 23, 2011

Kitava diet
http://www.cryonet.org/cgi-bin/dsp.cgi?msg=12909
June 1, 2011

Keratosis pilaris and teens
http://www.acneguide.com/acus_basics/like_acne/keratosis_pilaris.html
June 1, 2011

Is sugar toxic?

http://blog.seattlepi.com/timigustafsonrd/2011/04/
23/could-sugar-be-a-dangerous-toxin/
May 26, 2011

Sugar ages you

http://www.prevention.com/health/beauty/natural-
beauty/face-facts-about-
sugar/article/be6fc5bd0d115110VgnVCM1000001
3281eac____
May 26, 2011

LEAFY GREENS

A few years ago, after a cleansing fast, I began to crave salads. Soon greens became a staple of my diet. An ideal lunch or dinner included (and still includes) a few vegetables, and a bit of protein from fish, beans, eggs or chicken added to a bed of leafy greens, tossed with olive oil and balsamic vinegar, or fresh lemon juice. As I began making meals of salads, I began to eat less pasta and bread and fewer sugary sweets. The improved diet, along with other changes, helped my acne.

I didn't realize that leafy greens had a positive effect on my skin until I saw something in a magazine article about it. According to what I read, greens are "superfoods," high in antioxidants, like Vitamin E, that protect skin cells from free radical damage. I also learned that the vitamin A found in dark leafy greens like kale and spinach are great for clearing up acne and promoting skin repair. Vitamin A minimizes the production of sebum. This nutrient also strengthens the skin's protective tissue and helps to flush out toxins.

If you have severe acne, leafy greens alone won't clear it up. You'll have to make additional changes like those suggested earlier in the book. However, replacing less healthful foods with lots of leafy greens will help your skin and your overall health.

You can toss a bed of greens with all kinds of foods to create a healthy meal. Try not to add a salad dressing that contains high fructose corn syrup or sugar, though. Instead, consider drizzling with lemon or lime, balsamic or apple cider vinegar and olive oil.

Not a salad fan? Of course, you can cook leafy greens any way you wish. Try stir-frying some in coconut oil for an extra acne-fighting punch. Or try blending some spinach or kale into your favorite fruit smoothie. Adding just a small handful won't affect the taste, but you'll get the extra skin benefits.

References:

Leafy greens for acne
http://www.care2.com/greenliving/five-best-foods-for-skin.html#
May 5, 2011

http://www.brighthub.com/health/diet-nutrition/articles/42831.aspx#ixzz1LX9E9kjP
May 5, 2011

OMEGA 3s

Years ago, I began taking Omega 3's in combination with brushing the skin on my face; Both were suggested by my mother who felt she'd rid herself of adult acne with the combination. Serendipitously, the regimen not only helped to clear her acne, it also led to more youthful looking skin.

I can't say with certainty that the Omega 3's were a boon to my acne, because I was doing so many things, concurrently, to combat it, but I've recently come across a couple of articles that claim there is, indeed, a benefit.

One study suggests that adding Omega 3's to the diet leads to less sebum production and clearer pores. Another study found that taking Omega 3's led to fewer acne lesions among the participants of the study over a two-month period.

Despite the positive findings of these studies, as I scoured acne message boards, the results, according to posters, varied widely. Some people swore by taking Omega 3's, touting them as a miracle cure; some said it had no effect. And a few people said it made their acne worse.

It definitely did not make mine worse. I continue to take Omega 3's to this day and have been taking them regularly for about 12 years. While I wouldn't claim that they "cured" my acne, taking Omega 3's has undoubtedly made the quality of my skin better. When I don't take them, the skin is drier, its little lines are more visible, and the pores appear larger. When I take at least four, 1200mg capsules a day, my skin is plumper, suppler, and my pores are less noticeable.

If you're suffering from acne and you haven't tried fish oil capsules, I'd recommend them. How many per day depends on your size and your diet, and you should ask your doctor if they're appropriate for you. If you start taking the capsules on your own follow the recommendations on the bottle. Track your skin for a month to see if there's any improvement.

Be sure not to overdo it with the capsules, unless recommended by a doctor. If they seem to work for you and you want to enhance the benefits try adding foods containing Omega 3's to you diet. Some good choices are: salmon, sardines, walnuts, olive oil, and flaxseeds.

There are plenty of overall health benefits to taking Omega 3's. These benefits are primarily associated with their anti-inflammatory properties. Studies suggest they help alleviate depression in some people, they benefit the joints, the heart and, of course, the skin. Some of you will try them for your acne and get great results, and some of you will try them and not get the acne benefit you'd hoped for, but at the least you'll be doing something to benefit your overall health and beauty.

References:
http://www.worldhealth.net/news/omega-3_fatty_acids_and_acne/
May 19, 2011

http://www.goaskalice.columbia.edu/10733.html
May 19, 2011

http://www.webmd.com/diet/guide/good-fat-bad-fat-facts-about-omega-3
May 20, 2011

ZINC

Zinc, a metallic chemical element, is an essential mineral, found in every cell. Some people find that taking zinc supplements helps with acne management. While working on this book, as I researched some of the things I was already using, in order to learn more about why they worked, Zinc and its beneficial effect on acne came up repeatedly. I decided to look into it further, and I've begun taking the supplements myself.

I've long known that zinc was helpful to the skin. When I was a kid, my mother used zinc oxide, topically, to heal skin ailments—rashes, bites, and minor scratches and burns. As I began to read about zinc, I learned that studies have been conducted confirming that the mineral helps to heal the skin when taken internally as well.

According to the Office of Dietary Supplements zinc aids the immune system by helping it fight invading bacteria and viruses. It's an antioxidant, which means it protects the cells from damage caused by free radicals. This helps skin heal faster and stay healthy. And it also makes it ideal for restoring acne prone skin.

Dosage recommendations vary from 20mgs to 50mgs two times a day and some articles speak of taking up to 100mgs. I would recommend following the instructions on the bottle, to start. See if you notice a reduction of breakouts at whatever the recommended dosage is. If not, ask your doctor if it would be safe for you to try a little more. Don't take more than the recommended dosage without the advice of a medical professional, however, because too much zinc can be toxic. Some people have reported that on an empty stomach, zinc will cause vomiting, so take it with food and plenty of water. If you prefer food sources of zinc, you can find it in oysters, beef, poultry, dried beans and nuts, fortified cereals and dairy products.

Zinc for acne
http://www.mashmagazine.com/00april/aprilzinc.html

http://www.acnetohealth.com/zinc-gluconate-and-acne.html

http://www.umm.edu/altmed/articles/acne-000001.htm

http://www.ncbi.nlm.nih.gov/pubmed/10846252

http://ods.od.nih.gov/factsheets/Zinc-QuickFacts/

June 2, 2011

AEROBIC EXERCISE

It took me years to realize that exercise has beneficial effects on the skin. But if you think about it, it makes perfect sense. Exercise improves circulation. Your heart pumps faster which gets your blood flowing. If your blood is circulating well, it's bringing nutrients to the cells all over your body, including those in your skin.

Exercise also causes us to perspire. One of the ways the body expels toxins is through perspiration. Your pores get a bit of a flushing, as sweat expels what's inside those pores.

According to WebMD, the most pronounced effects of exercise are on acne-prone skin.
Why? Because exercise reduces the production of testosterone related hormones as it reduces stress.

Stress often leads to breakouts, because when we're stressed our adrenal glands produce hormones like DHEA and DHT, which are testosterone related and contribute to breakouts. Exercise quiets the adrenals, helping to calm acne.

Exercise helps to make breakouts less frequent and less severe. One of the things dermatologists recommend is that you hydrate (preferably with water) prior to exercise. When you're properly hydrated this helps circulation, and when you exercise and get your blood flowing, the blood can then transport nutrients around the body and to your skin.

David Goldberg, a dermatologist quoted on WebMD says: "The better your circulation, which is something aerobic exercise can improve, the more effectively toxins are removed. The better and healthier your skin will not only be, but also look."

The type of exercise you do is up to you, but it should be something that gets your heart rate up and something that causes you to sweat. I walk regularly around a track, but I find stair climbing (regular steps in a building) gives me the best clear-skin results. Two or three times a week, for 20 to 30 minutes at a time, I hike up and down seven flights of stairs in a nearby parking structure. In just a few minutes I work up a sweat and get my blood pumping.

Do whatever aerobic exercise you enjoy and can commit to doing on a regular basis. Use caution though; try not to wear makeup or oily hair-care products when you work out. Oil from hair products can drip down onto your skin when you perspire and products containing comedogenic ingredients can cause breakouts. Be sure that any makeup you use while exercising is oil-free and non-comedogenic.

Wash immediately after exercise.

This might seem like obvious or even condescending advice. I apologize if so, but some people don't realize the importance of the habit of washing immediately after exercise in controlling acne.

Exercise is great for your skin, because the increased blood flow brings nutrients to the tissues, and sweating releases toxins, but if you're acne prone allowing the toxins and bacteria to sit on your skin is *not* going to be good. Your sweat attracts bacteria, and damp sweaty clothes create an ideal environment for the bacteria to flourish. Do yourself a favor and get out of those clothes, and wash up as quickly as possible. Don't give bacteria a chance to get into your pores and cause breakouts.

References:

Exercise and benefit to acne prone skin

http://www.webmd.com/skin-problems-and-treatments/acne/features/exercise-your-body-your-skin

http://www.acne-advice.com/articles/exercise/index.shtml
April 26, 2011

Control bacteria after exercise
http://www.acne-advice.com/articles/exercise/index.shtml
May 25, 2011

Shower immediately after exercise
http://www.acneskintreatment.org/exercise-and-acne.htm
June 3, 2011

SKIN BRUSHING

I'm fairly new to dry skin brushing, but I've become a quick convert. After doing it fairly consistently for four weeks now, my skin is smooth, soft and vibrant.

The skin is an organ, our largest organ, and the skin is one of the pathways through which our body sheds toxins. When we brush our skin we slough off dead skin cells and toxins along with them.

You may be wondering yeah, great, but is skin brushing going to cure my acne? *Cure it,* not exactly. BUT, there *are* helpful benefits to skin brushing, including improved circulation; stimulating blood flow to the surface of the skin (which brings nutrients to it), stimulating the lymphatic system, and toxin removal. While these things alone won't eradicate acne, they will work in concert with other natural remedies to promote healthier skin.

One of the things skin brushing advocates mention repeatedly is how it benefits the lymphatic system. Most of you probably understand what better blood circulation is, but you may not be as familiar with the lymphatic system, what it does, and how it relates to the skin. The lymphatic system is responsible for:

a) balancing fluids— after the cells are bathed with needed nutrients, the lymphatic system drains excess fluid from the tissues as lymph,
b) removing undesirable substances from the blood,

c) assimilating fats not previously absorbed by the small intestines.

The lymphatic system is an important defense and filtration system. Unlike the circulatory system, lymph is not pumped around the body with the aid of the heart; it depends upon the movement of muscles, breathing and gravity. Skin brushing is an additional way the lymphatic system can be assisted.

Don't be confused and use the brush you use on your body to brush your face. I'm going to discuss brushing the face, but right now, we're focusing on the rest of the body.

Proponents of skin brushing advise that we brush (with a natural bristle skin brush) prior to a shower or hot bath and some advise brushing prior to exercise. It's recommended that we brush from the soles of the feet all the way to the neck, always brushing toward the heart. Avoid brushing over bruises, rashes or cuts.

Use can use straight and circular motions from the bottom of the feet, up the legs and over hips, thighs and buttocks brushing up toward the heart. Go over the abdomen and lower back, when you reach the upper chest, continue, but brush down toward the heart, rather than up toward the head. From the shoulder, to the upper arm, brush down and inward, toward the chest. On the hands and lower arm, brush up and in toward the chest. On the upper back, brush down.

At first, go lightly, especially in spots where your skin is sensitive. As you keep brushing regularly, your skin should be able to tolerate more pressure and you'll begin to experience the benefits of exfoliation, toxin removal and better blood flow to the skin, which will leave it softer, smoother and more radiant.

After your shower or bath, be sure to moisturize your skin with a good quality lotion. I prefer lotions without chemical additives, so I recommend pure coconut oil, or castor oil.

References:

Skin brushing
http://www.jashbotanicals.com/articles/skin_brushing.html

Benefits of skin brushing
http://www.skin-care.becomegorgeous.com/perfect_skin/dry_skin_brushing_benefits-1710.html
April 26, 2011

Lymphatic system
http://www.anatomy.tv/StudyGuides/StudyGuide.aspx?guideid=20&nextID=16&maxID=0&customer=primal
April 26, 2011

BRUSH YOUR FACE

Okay, I *could* just have said, "exfoliate" your face, because that's the anti-acne benefit of "brushing" your face.

Years ago, my mother began brushing her face with a toothbrush to exfoliate and clean her pores. She started doing this after seeing an aesthetician who gave her a facial that began with a skin brushing. Mom figured a toothbrush (obviously not the same one she used on her teeth) would give similar results to the face brush the facialist had used.

It was true; the brushing did exfoliate and help her keep her pores clear. The unexpected, added benefit was that her fine lines and wrinkles were minimized. Though this isn't an anti-aging book, I've decided to recommend the face brushing for acne and if you do it and it helps you look younger, lucky you.

Put whatever cleanser you choose on the brush, wet the face first. It might help to open your pores with a warm washcloth, and then brush all the areas of your face in circular motions. I like to start at the sides of the mouth, moving up to the cheeks, very gently around the eyes, then onto the forehead and finally the nose and chin. At first you should scrub gently. Of course, you never want to scrub so hard that you break the skin. Brush just firmly enough to gently exfoliate. It's okay if your face is a bit red when you finish. The redness should subside within a few minutes. If it doesn't, scrub more gently the next time. Your skin will eventually build up a tolerance to the exfoliation, and the redness will be less pronounced and dissipate more quickly.

Of course you can exfoliate with exfoliating creams, a buff puff, a rough washcloth, or whatever you like. My preference is a soft to medium bristle toothbrush, because in addition to the exfoliation, the brushing action seems to give the skin and underlying tissues a workout akin to doing facial exercises.

Brushing will sweep dead skin cells off the surface of the skin, helping to prevent clogged pores that can lead to break outs. It also leaves the skin in a state that allows the products you're using to penetrate the skin more easily, and thus work more effectively.

The Clarisonic Face Brush is a popular, albeit expensive, product that many acne sufferers swear by. It was inspired by The Clarisonic Electric Toothbrush. In my experience, you can get equivalent results with a regular toothbrush. Exfoliation will benefit your skin no matter how you achieve it.

References:

Electric toothbrush for acne
http://www.acne.org/messageboard/TOOTH-BRUSH-METHOD-SMOOT-t211818.html
May 25, 2011

USE A NEW WASHCLOTH DAILY

When I was a kid, my mother, a depression era child, was very stingy with things like washcloths and toothbrushes. I think I had the same toothbrush from about age 7—12! Laundry was done only every 10 days or so. I used the same washcloth every day. This is the bane of acne

Acne causing bacteria can build up on a stale, damp washcloth. If you wipe your face with a wet washcloth and either Propionibacterium Acnes or Staphylococcus Aures (bacteria known to cause acne) are on your skin, you'll transfer them to the cloth. A damp washcloth provides an ideal environment for bacteria to thrive. What happens when you go to use that cloth again and you wipe your face with it? You transfer more bacteria back to your skin!

 My advice is to buy a large pack of washcloths and have a small basket or hamper in your bathroom where you can toss one in each day. That way you won't have to do laundry too often, but you'll make sure not to reintroduce bacteria to your skin over and over with a stale washcloth. When you wash your washcloths, do so in hot water, which will help kill the bacteria.

If you use a buff puff or a face brush, it's a good idea to wash in hot water frequently, or spray it regularly with vinegar, or alcohol, or some kind of antibacterial spray.

References:

Change washcloths frequently
Ciraldo, Loretta. *6 Weeks to Sensational Skin*, (New York: Rodale, 2006.) 14, 102.

http://www.acne-ltd.com/lifestyle.php3
June 1, 2011

CHANGE PILLOW CASES FREQUENTLY

If you sleep on your side or on your stomach, your face probably presses into your pillow.

The oils from your skin and dead skin cells can slough off onto the pillowcase and with them, dust and dirt from the air, and bacteria from your own skin, hair and the environment. If your skin is particularly oily and you regularly end up on your face while you sleep, I'd recommend changing the pillowcases as often as every day, if possible. At the least, change them twice a week and you'll help reduce the amount of bacteria your skin comes into contact with.

When you wash your pillowcases, the detergent you use can also aggravate sensitive skin. If so, do an extra rinse with hot water, to be sure to get the detergent residue out of the fabric. You can also try washing your pillowcases in vinegar and baking soda rather than regular detergent. This combination will kill bacteria, but it's mild enough that it should not irritate sensitive skin.

I recommend washing your pillows regularly also. Did you know you could wash pillows? It never occurred to me until fairly recently. I used to just throw them out once they were too dirty to look at anymore. But unless they're feather filled, pillows can be washed in the washing machine and dried in the dryer. If you suffer from acne, I recommend that you do this at least once every couple of months or more frequently. Dust mites, dead skin and oils collect in our pillows and though your pillowcase covers it, it can be helpful to keep the pillow itself clean as well.

References:

Change pillow case to prevent acne
http://www.fitsugar.com/Change-Pillow-Case-Regularly-Prevent-Acne-Outbreaks-1708461

http://www.emaxhealth.com/1506/73/33903/change-pillowcase-often-prevent-acne-skin-problems.html
June 1, 2011

DISINFECT PHONES FREQUENTLY

When I speak on the phone a lot I notice that I tend to develop pimples around my mouth and chin area where the phone rests. As the phone rubs onto my face, any dirt, dust, germs or oils on the phone mix with the oils, bacteria, and dirt on my face. Additionally, saliva and breath create a moist environment, perfect for bacteria to flourish. If the phone is pressed on my face long enough, there's added gunk due to any perspiration and friction caused by the phone rubbing on my skin. There's actually a name for this: "Acne Mechanica," which is defined as a form of acne cause by heat, covered skin and repetitive friction.

Clean your phone off with anti-bacterial wipes or alcohol frequently. If you work at a job wherein you must hold the phone to your face, keep some wipes nearby and wipe the phone before you use it.

References:

Phone acne?
http://www.ienhance.com/articles/skin/adult-acne
May 17, 2011

Acne mechanica (acne caused by friction)
http://www.lifescript.com/Health/Conditions/Skin/
Battling_Grown-Up_Breakouts.aspx
May 17, 2011

Acne mechanica

http://www.skincarephysicians.com/acnenet/article
_acnemechanica.html
May 17, 2011

AVOID OIL-BASED PRODUCTS AND MAKEUP

I can't stress this enough for people with acne prone skin. The tendency is, especially if you're a woman, to cover up pimples with makeup. But if no one tells you that oil-based makeup clogs your pores and causes breakouts, you will probably just think you have bad skin and you'll keep piling on foundation to cover those unsightly zits, without realizing you're creating more of them as you strive to hide them. Stop using any makeup or cover up that contains any kind of oil.

Mineral powder makeup is a better choice, because it doesn't clog your pores. You can also use water-based foundations if you prefer a more traditional kind of coverage.

Stop using moisturizer that contains mineral oil, or petroleum, or other kinds of oils, unless the oils in the product are specified to be types that do not clog pores (non-comedogenic). As I've mentioned, I used to douse my skin with Vitamin E oil when I was younger, thinking it was good for my acne, because vitamin E is supposed to be healing. I didn't realize that it was actually clogging my pores and creating more acne, not healing it.

There *are* oils that acne prone people can use, but read the labels and if you aren't sure, it's best to avoid them.

I have a friend, Monique, who suffered with moderate acne. She was using oil-based makeup without realizing that it was clogging her pores. Once she stopped the makeup, her skin cleared up completely. Now it's glowing and gorgeous. According to her, omitting the oil-based foundation was the *only* change she made, and her skin was transformed.

If you're using an oil-based foundation and suffering from acne, you might be surprised by how well your skin will respond when you cut it out.

Also, be careful of any hair care products containing oily ingredients. Even if you don't put them on your face they can seep down onto your skin when you're overheated or when you're sleeping.

References:

Oil-based makeup worsens acne
http://articles.baltimoresun.com/1994-03-08/features/1994067145_1_acne-makeup-to-cover-hair-oil
May 17, 2011

Don't use oil-based makeup
http://www.joys-of-lavender.com/acne.html
June 1, 201

VISUALIZATION

You may be thinking, *visualization? What?! How could THAT possibly benefit acne? Please.*

But hear me out. Thoughts are so powerful. If you're constantly thinking about your acne and how terrible it looks, you're reinforcing that image of yourself. You may not be *consciously* thinking these thoughts; you may not intend to be doing it; but if you're upset about your acne, feeling terrible about it, then your emotions are engaged and your subconscious is likely to be involved, too, which only helps to keep your energy stuck in a place where you're breaking out and feeling bad.

I know from my own experience that I felt ugly and frustrated when my acne was as its worst. It consumed my sense of self until I almost felt as if I *was* the acne. You may not be as bad as that, but if your self-esteem is suffering, then visualization can help you.

Make some time to get quiet.
Sit comfortably and close your eyes.
Breathe deeply and slowly, calming your body.
It's been suggested that beginning with the thought of something that makes you happy and/or grateful, enhances the effects of the meditation.
When you feel good, begin to picture your skin being flawless. If it's just your face picture that, or if you prefer, see your whole body with clear, glowing skin.

See yourself smiling, feeling great that your skin looks so radiant, healthy and clear.

You may want to say some affirmations to yourself. For example: *My skin is clear and glowing.* Or, *Thank you for my healthy, clear skin.* Or, *My skin is flawless from head to toe.*

Notice that the affirmations are in the present tense. That's because you are trying to create what you're saying as if it's true now. It will feel silly and false at first, if you're not used to it. But if you were to say, "I wish I had clear skin," that isn't as powerful. Or if you were to say, "One day I'll have clear skin," that's not great either, because you're affirming that it's always in the future. We want to create it in the *now*.

Even though it will feel like you're lying, or crazy, stick with it. Eventually your mind will click in and know how to use it.

Sit and picture yourself with clear skin and feel great about it, for at least 10 minutes, while saying your affirmation. If you can do it longer, that would be great. Try to do it for at least 10 minutes every day.

When you finish your visualization and go on with the rest of your day, occasionally say the affirmation again, and if convenient, recall the image of yourself with your pristine, clear skin. Eventually, you'll begin to change the image of yourself, which will help you make the transformation.

Years ago, before I learned about natural remedies for acne, I did a similar meditation for a while. Within about 10 days, I was led to the friend who told me about the aloe vera juice and acidophilus, which I mentioned earlier. My skin began to clear up and I've kept it pretty clear since. It was the information I needed to make a real change. When you being to visualize what you want, you draw things to you to help you make it happen.

References:

Visualization for acne
http://www.acne.org/visualization.php

http://www.20daypersuasion.com/free-acne-treatment2.htm
June 4, 2011

A PLAN TO GET STARTED

So, now that I've given you all this information, you may be feeling that it's too much to assimilate and follow. You're probably wondering, *where do I begin?* Start here:

SHOPPING LIST

I've recommended things that are not on this list and you can and should try them, but first let's try the following:

1. Aloe Vera Juice- unsweetened.
You can find good brands at Trader Joe's or Walmart. It should cost around $8. If you can't get it there, look for it online. Be sure there are no added sugars.

2. Pure aloe vera gel, preferably from the plant. You can buy aloe plants at a garden store, or nursery, or online. You can buy commercial aloe vera gel at drug stores, or places where they sell natural product, or online.

3. Green Tea
You can find it at most supermarkets. Prices vary, but inexpensive varieties should have the benefits we want, so they're fine. The low-cost varieties have 100 bags for about $3.50.

4. Baking Soda
You can find it in drugs stores and grocery stores for about $1 a pound or less.

5. Organic, unfiltered Apple Cider Vinegar
Trader Joe's carries its own brand. It's under $3.
Braggs is another good brand, available in health food
stores or online.

6. Virgin Coconut Oil
Whole Foods carries it. Some Ralphs Grocery Stores
carry it as well. It can be a bit pricey. I prefer to buy it
on Amazon.com and can usually find the 54oz size
for between $25 and $30.

7. Omega 3 Fish Oil Capsules
Available in drug stores. A good bottle of 100
capsules might run you $10--$15.

8. Plain, Unsweetened Yogurt
Found in any grocery store. Be sure to buy kinds with
active yogurt cultures, especially, *acidophilus.* A
32oz. container runs between $2--$5 depending upon
the brand. Even though milk fat can cause some of us
to break out, yogurt usually helps acne. I use lowfat
or nonfat varieties, but regular yogurt should be fine,
too. If you try the regular and suspect that it causes a
breakout, switch to nonfat and see if that makes a
difference.

9. Fresh Leafy Greens
You can use spinach, Kale, Romaine lettuce, or
whatever type you prefer. These are generally about
$1--$2 a bunch.

Here's how I recommend using these 9 things:

Morning:

Wash your face with BAKING SODA, mixed with water, as per instructions in the chapter. Afterwards, use a toner of ORGANIC APPLE CIDER VINEGAR and equal parts water, applied with a cotton ball over the face. Follow with about a half-teaspoon of COCONUT OIL melted in the hands and spread over the entire face. Pat off excess with a tissue or paper towel. Follow with non-comedogenic sunscreen.

With breakfast, drink two cups of GREEN TEA and eat a cup of PLAIN, UNSWEETENED YOGURT. If you can't stomach the yogurt with nothing in it, try adding some berries and/or chopped almonds or walnuts to it.

You can eat other things, too, this isn't a diet plan, but avoid high glycemic index foods containing sugar or white flour. Avoid donuts, bagels and sugary cereals. Try whole grain cereals, or eggs instead.

After breakfast take your OMEGA 3s. Consult your doctor for the proper amount for you. I take two each morning and evening.

At Lunch and Dinner:

Include some LEAFY GREENS with your meals. Consider a salad tossed with chicken or fish. If you use salad dressing, please avoid those with added sugar. Instead try olive oil mixed with coconut oil and APPLE CIDER VINEGAR, or olive oil/COCONUT OIL and lemon juice. The reason I suggest mixing the olive oil with coconut oil is that coconut oil hardens at temperatures below 76 degrees and it won't pour over salad unless you mix it with olive oil, which helps liquefy it.

Sometime before or after dinner, drink a glass of ALOE VERA JUICE. Start with 4oz. Build up to at least 8oz.

Before bed:

Take Omega 3s again.

Wash your face with BAKING SODA
Tone with APPLE CIDER VINEGAR mixed with equal parts water. Leave on the skin.
Moisturize with COCONUT OIL, pat off excess with tissue or a cloth.

A few times a week, apply PLAIN YOGURT to clean skin and allow to dry before washing off, OR leave on overnight (instead of coconut oil) and wash off in the morning.

If you have access to an aloe vera plant, apply pure the gel to the face (as per instructions in the chapter) two or three times per week. You can also use commercial aloe vera gel. Put it on at night, before the coconut oil, (applying the coconut oil on top of the gel after it dries) or just use the on its own.

Before sleep: Affirm that your skin is smooth and blemish free, then close your eyes and picture it that way.

A few other things to try right away:

1. Omit any oil-based creams or cosmetics.
2. Do some aerobic exercise daily, if possible. No less than 4 times per week. Get your heart rate up and work up a sweat. Wash up right after your workout.
3. If you use a washcloth, change it daily.
4. Change your pillowcases frequently.
5. Drink more water.
6. Limit, or preferably eliminate sugar, white flour, and white rice from your diet.

These suggestions are just a start. You'll have to use trial and error to find what works for you, or what doesn't. If the coconut oil doesn't seem to help, give castor oil, neem, or tea tree oil a try. In fact, even with the coconut oil, you can use neem or tea tree oil to dab on individual lesions.

If the aloe vera juice doesn't feel good, consider the instructions for drinking apple cider vinegar and water, or drink more green tea. Or if you don't like green tea, try white tea. Do be sure to give the dietary suggestions at least a few days to a week to work, unless, of course, you have an adverse reaction, in which case you should discontinue immediately.

CLOSING

It's been a great pleasure sharing this information with you. I hope you've found something within these pages helpful in your pursuit of acne-free skin. My goal has been to suggest things that are healthful, and that can be incorporated into your lifestyle safely, and beneficially, for long periods of time, unlike some medically prescribed acne cures that can cause unpleasant side effects, or be detrimental to use long term.

I know first hand how difficult dealing with acne can be. Think of this book as a hug from someone who understands and cares. My wish is that you attain the clear, glowing and vibrant skin you want, so that you can shine in the world confidently and give your best in all endeavors.

Warmly,

Toni Ann

INTERVIEWS

The following section contains a series of interviews with people who are managing adult acne. I'm including these, because they provide an additional perspective and advice that differs, in some ways, from what I've recommended. Some of you may find the alternatives helpful. My goal with this book is not to insist upon *my* way, but rather to provide information that leads to the best result for the reader. I hope you find something helpful here.

MONIQUE MATTHEWS

When did you realize that you had acne prone skin?

I was in high school – junior year, I think. I would get a huge, red ugly pimple on my nose. My mom would laugh, saying that it was a clear indication that I was on my period. I was mortified.

I started reading Seventeen magazine, for no one in my family was into skin care. And, they had ads all the time about acne, so I figured they were experts. I began to realize that I generally got acne in the T-zone. I thought I had combination skin because that's what the articles and illustrations said. It wasn't until I was fresh out of college that I learned that my skin was not combination, but oily. I had an HMO plan and I really didn't know how to choose a doctor, so I chose a dermatologist in Beverly Hills because I figured he was good. He recommended Retin A, but I never used it. I'd had an earlier experience in high school when my mom gave me some of her Retin A and it caused more outbreaks. I realize that it was too strong.

Did you see a dermatologist? If so, was medication prescribed? What were the results?

I did not see a dermatologist at the time of my initial outbreak. Somehow, given my background and my family's focus on "natural beauty," (which meant no makeup not even lipstick) I felt ashamed to care about my skin. It meant that I was vain, and I didn't want to be that, so I self-treated via Seventeen magazine and other teen 'zines.

What dietary changes, if any, did you make in an effort to control your acne?

My major problems with acne came from not recognizing my skin type and not using the right type of skin cleaner. I'd use Ivory or Noxzema. I have always been active and generally considerate of food choices, so I don't believe I've had a significant amount of dietary changes.

Did you make any non-dietary changes to your lifestyle in order to control acne?

My non-dietary changes were not really conscious choices. As I previously mentioned, I grew up in an environment where I felt shamed for focusing on my skin, as if it meant that I was superficial and/or siddity. My choice to lead an active lifestyle, take multi-vitamins and peruse health and fitness magazines and books resulted from a plethora of chronic diseases that plagued my immediate family. I was more focused on avoiding the illnesses that many in my family experienced: heart disease, lung disease and high blood pressure among others. Achieving clear skin, as a result of exercise and diet, was a happy side effect, not a conscious motivation.

What do you think causes the kind of acne you have? Are there any specific triggers you can point to?

I have extremely sensitive and delicate skin. I have to avoid any product that's made for "normal" skin, not hypoallergenic nor non-comodogenic.

In regards to diet, I expect a breakout if I eat something that I normally do not, such as fried chicken, mass amounts of fast food, and oily foods.

I also do my best to avoid strong spirits. While I do drink red wine, specifically Pinot Noir because it's the highest in Resveratrol, I try to restrict my intake of anything that is 80 proof or higher. Scotch, for example, breaks me out. Other strong spirits such as vodka and rum do not break me out, but make my skin dull and flat, if I consume a significant amount (3 or more drinks).

Do you take medication or use any types of drugs to treat your acne now? If so, which ones?

I take a daily multi-vitamin. Besides that, I do not take any other drugs, prescription or otherwise.

As I've previously mentioned, my clear skin results largely from my focus on health and nutrition. I come from a family plagued with chronic illness, and I made a decision at age nine that things would be different from me. My father and I would often go on weekly father/daughter dates. We'd always go to 86th Street and 3rd Avenue in New York, because they had great movie theaters, Barnes and Noble and a really cool toy store. They also had a GNC. We went in there when I was ten and I began taking my first supplement, black strap molasses, which is high in iron to strengthen my blood and give me energy.

I avoid most white food products – rice, sugar, and the like. I eat spinach nearly every day. I avoid oils and products cooked in oil that are high in unhealthy saturated fats. I regularly cook and eat with olive oil, grape seed oil, and I've recently begun experimenting with coconut oil, thanks to Toni Ann.

There are times when I use flaxseed oil, specifically as a complement to a protein rich meal of egg whites, tomatoes, chicken and feta cheese for breakfast.

I have also had times when I began my morning with a glass of hot water with lemon. Most recently, the first thing I consume when I wake up in the morning directly after 8 – 12 ounces of water is a "hot tea" consisting of two tablespoons of apple cider vinegar and one tablespoon of honey in 8 ounces of filtered, hot water.

I also use organic, extra-virgin coconut oil on my body and face and ingest one teaspoon, daily.

Do you exercise? If so, what do you do, and do you think it has any effect on your skin?

I exercise three to four times a week. I remember when I was training for the Los Angeles marathon that there was a slogan at Gold's Gym – Hollywood that said, "Endorphins are cheaper than Prozac." I'd recently graduated from UCLA Film School and was embarking on an often-elusive career in the Entertainment Industry as a writer. Working out kept me sane, focused and provided a healthy outlet for any neurosis I might have.

I completed two triathlons in 2010, which was fantastic for my body and my sense of self. Often when I work out, I try to imagine something that I think is impossible and I go for it. I realize that if I can complete the impossible, anything is possible.

I believe that working out eliminates toxins as well as eliminating any potential for stress-based acne to rear its ugly head.

When your skin has been its best what were you doing?

When my skin is operating at its best, it often means that I am focused, happy and on track with my life, relationship and career goals. As I mentioned, for me, healthy skin is a great byproduct of putting my health first.

What advice can you share with other acne sufferers?

Having healthy clean skin is a right and privilege that everyone should have. Pursuing it does not make one vain or superficial; it's a direct result of honoring the vessel you've been given to use on this planet. It also is not expensive. There are simple, healthy options that you can employ to achieve optimal skin care.

Monique N. Matthews is a Los Angeles based writer/director. Prior to filmmaking, she was an entertainment journalist and managing editor of a national hip-hop magazine. She has written for several studios, worked with a variety of production companies and has received several accolades including *Daily Variety's* "10 Writers to Watch" and *Filmmaker* magazine's "25 New Faces of Independent Film." Monique was also selected to participate in Film Independent's prestigious Directors and Writers Labs. In 2006, she wrote and directed "It Looks Just Like You," an awareness commercial about breast cancer that received a million dollars in free advertising to run on BET. Monique is also an associate professor at Santa Monica College, where she serves in several departments, including English, Communication and Film Studies.

http://web.me.com/moniquenmatthews

LEONARD CHANG

When did you discover that you had acne prone skin?

In high school, when I began to have minor but persistent breakouts. My mother has dealt with adult acne, as has my older brother, so I knew I was predisposed to this.

Did you see a dermatologist? If so, was medication prescribed? What were the results?

No dermatologist, but I began using over-the-counter medication, such as lotions with Benzoyl Peroxide or salicylic acid. I had erratic results. Sometimes it worked, sometimes it didn't, and it often dried out my skin.

What dietary changes, if any, did you make in an effort to control your acne?

When I was younger I didn't make any dietary changes. Lately I've been more aware of how my diet affects my skin, so the most recent change, based on the advice of this book, was the introduction of aloe vera juice.

Did you make any non-dietary changes to your lifestyle in order to control acne?

I'm more aware of the kinds of soaps and lotions I use on my face. I've found that extra virgin food-grade coconut oil is better than most commercial moisturizers, without any deleterious effects. I avoid lotions with too many fragrances and unfamiliar chemicals and ingredients.

What do you think causes the kind of acne you have? Are there any specific triggers you can point to?

Stress seems to trigger it. Cold, dry weather also occasionally seems to cause breakouts. Although now I suspect I may have been using acne-inducing lotions to compensate for the dry weather, and it was these, not the weather, that was causing the acne.

Do you take medication or use any types of drugs to treat your acne now? If so, which ones?

I still occasionally use an over-the-counter cream with Benzoyl Peroxide, as well as a green tea astringent.

Do you use any kinds of food or supplements to control your acne? If so, what do you use?

Just aloe vera juice, although now, because of this book, I've learned more about yogurt and green tea, and have been more consistent in having these with the specific goal of helping my skin.

Do you exercise? If so, what do you do, and do you think it has any effect on your skin?

I exercise everyday -- usually at the gym, often running/hiking, or rock climbing -- and I can't be sure whether or not it has an effect on my skin because I've been doing this since I was a young kid. I suspect it helps, especially the outdoor activity like running and hiking. The sweating, the blood flow and then the cleaning afterwards all seems to contribute to better skin.

When your skin has been its best what were you doing?

Either living in Jamaica, when I was with the Peace Corps, or vacationing in Hawaii. The sun, sea and being outdoors in warm, tropical weather seems to be the best for my skin.

What advice can you share with other acne sufferers?

Diet is much more important than I realized, and I think the aloe vera juice helps quite a bit. Paying more attention to the ingredients in lotions and soaps, and trying to stay as natural as possible definitely has helped my skin.

Leonard Chang is a novelist, and television writer trying to live a low-stress life in Santa Monica, California.

LISA M. PITT

When did you discover that you had acne prone skin?

It started at puberty with me. My skin broke out so bad that my mom took me to the doctor. It was my pediatrician that recommended Aveeno Soap over 30 years ago. I still use Aveeno Soap today and find it the most effective product for cleansing and healing my acne prone skin. By college, I noticed I would have large and small pimples breakout on my forehead, nose and chin. My acne would flare up during my menstrual cycle and just never seemed to go away. As I grew into my 20s, 30s, and 40s, I realized that I was still struggling with acne as other adults around me appeared to have pimple free skin.

Did you see a dermatologist? If so, was medication prescribed? What were the results?

I have gone to dermatologists over the years for treatments. The most recent (in my 40s) prescribed Epiduo (adapalene and benzoyl peroxide) after a particular harrowing period where I couldn't seem to get my breakouts under control. She also recommended a salicylic acid face wash so I used a Neutrogena brand. Over a two-year period, I used a normal strength peroxide face wash - an over the counter brand sold only at my health care provider's pharmacy. I mixed or alternated the facial washing products and applied prescription grade medication once a day. The combination of products worked but I found them to be extremely drying. Once the acne breakouts became less severe, I switched back to my normal cleansing routine.

What dietary changes, if any, did you make in an effort to control your acne?

In college, I realized my skin would clear up if I drank unusually large amounts of water. I became so used to ingesting large amounts of water that I could consume almost an entire gallon in continuous gulps. Many times it is not practical to drink that much water (and I wouldn't recommend it unless a bathroom is in reasonable proximity for several hours). Eliminating greasy foods was recommended but I found this difficult to do in my 20s as I seemed to live off of potato chips. In all, I would definitely attribute increased water intake to helping control my adult acne.

Did you make any non-dietary changes to your lifestyle in order to control acne?

Well I have on several occasions developed an eye twitch from lack of sleep. I do notice that if I get more rest, my skin looks and feels better. Also, during bad breakouts, I would not use oil on my hair, or I'd wipe my hairline with an astringent, as well as change my pillowcases. I don't know that these modifications reduced the acne on my face but they certainly didn't make it worse.

What do you think causes the kind of acne you have? Are there any specific triggers you can point to?

I have very oily, thick skin that is easily susceptible to clogging. For instance, I had a little skin nodule on my eyelid for many years. The various doctors that examined it speculated that it was an over active or infected cell derived from having oily skin. I tend to break out less on my cheeks but my pores are bigger in those areas. I definitely know that my hormonal cycle affects my breakouts. There are other triggers that probably exacerbate my acne flair ups like stress and/or oily hair, skin and food products.

Overall I suspect that my skin is acne prone whether triggers are present or not. I know the literature differentiates teenage acne, which tends to cover the forehead, nose, cheeks, and chin, from adult acne, which presents around the mouth, chin and jawline. My face actually continues to break out in all those places without any regard for age. At this stage in my life, acne and I are as one but I just have the upper hand.

Do you take medication or use any types of drugs to treat your acne now? If so, which ones?

I don't take oral medication because of the associated risks. I simply use topical prescriptions when needed.

Do you use any kinds of food or supplements to control your acne? If so, what do you use?

I am very suspect of greasy foods so I tend to watch it in this area when I can. Also, I take collagen, and acidophilus regularly, and multivitamins or vitamin E for periods of time.

Do you exercise? If so, what do you do, and do you think it has any effect on your skin?

Yes I exercise a lot which means I sweat a great deal. I also use the hot dry sauna on a regular basis to open my pores, and I prefer a wet sauna if available. I consider the sauna part of my exercise routine.

When your skin has been its best what were you doing?

Sleeping well, eating wholesome foods, drinking LOTS of water, and exercising until I work up a sweat.

What advice can you share with other acne sufferers?

Don't give up! It took me a long time to find the right mix of products and understand my breakout cycles. Not everything advertised to cure acne will work. Also, if something is damaging skin because it's too harsh, stop using it. I literally have scarred my skin using scrubs that are way too abrasive. There are too many products out there to keep using those that provide minimal results. Keep track of what works and add the right mix of solutions to your skin care regimen. Mine started with a little beige bar of Aveeno soap decades ago, and continues to evolve.

Lisa M. Pitt is the founder of Forty Plus Buffed, a website dedicated to maturing adults interested in health, diet, fitness and anti-aging. As a mother of three young children, Lisa attributes her youthful appearance and physique to life-long athleticism. She is an advocate for good nutrition, exercise, anti-aging skin techniques and natural hair care. In her work as a fitness instructor, she has designed workout programs for all fitness levels. Lisa received her MBA from University of California, and Bachelor of Arts degree from Yale University. She maintains an active lifestyle and enjoys racquetball, basketball, tennis, rock climbing, triathlon training (run/swim/bike), Pilates, yoga, step aerobics, weight lifting, kickboxing, boxing, and dance (Latin/hip hop/ballet/contemporary/jazz/belly dancing).

www.fortyplusbuffed.com

DANIELLE STALLINGS

When did you discover that you had acne prone skin?

I had acne long before I understood that I had "acne prone skin." I didn't put 2+2 together for many years. I thought it was just unlucky and didn't realize there was a cause.

Did you see a dermatologist? If so, was medication prescribed? What were the results?

I've been to several dermatologists over the years. I don't do well on antibiotics and am against taking them long term, on principle, so I settled with a physician who didn't try to push the antibiotics on me like most of them do and she just let me use Retin A. Retin A worked OK but it never prevented break outs. It only helped to clear them up and I always ended up with peeling skin.

What dietary changes, if any, did you make in an effort to control your acne?

I made some dietary changes this year as a result of other health issues and discovered that my acne went away when I eliminated dairy, gluten, caffeine and sugar. Oddly enough I probably eat more fat than ever (since giving up those other things) but it seems to have no effect on my acne. I always thought eating fat/oil was one of the principle causes of acne. I guess not... at least for me. I need to mention though that I'm not really eating animal fat (no meat or dairy). I'm eating more nuts and tortilla chips... they just seem to satiate me now that I've given up gluten.

Did you make any non-dietary changes to your lifestyle in order to control acne?

I bought some glycolic acid products that my dermatologist sells but I think it's the diet change that got rid of my acne and not those cosmetic products.

What do you think causes the kind of acne you have? Are there any specific triggers you can point to?

I think it's clearly 95% diet, in my case. I do break out just a little when I wear sunscreen (and it's a "natural" sunscreen ironically). But otherwise I don't break out anymore, not even when I wear makeup, which used to be a big problem for me. In fact, I don't need to wear base anymore because I have nothing to cover up! I've pretty much given up using base and only wear eye makeup now.

Do you take medication or use any types of drugs to treat your acne now? If so, which ones?

Not really. I have a big tube of Retin A in the drawer that I bought from a Canadian pharmacy because my insurance wouldn't cover it. It just sits there now. I use the glycolic toner about 2-3 times a week, but even forget to use it. It's pretty amazing...

Do you use any kinds of food or supplements to

control your acne? If so, what do you use?

No. Now that I've eliminated gluten, dairy, sweets and caffeine I don't see any effects on my skin from other foods or supplements. I do buy purified water and sometimes splurge on the super "alkaline" water but don't really know if that's made a difference for my skin.

Do you exercise? If so, what do you do, and do you think it has any effect on your skin?

I'm exercising haphazardly right now. Bike, pilates, stretching, a little yoga. I can't say that I really notice a difference. (Except for when I bike and use that "natural" sunscreen that makes me break out.)

When your skin has been its best what were you doing?

Eating raw/vegan. I did that for 6 weeks straight one time and the health effects were astounding. I even got rid of my cellulite.

What advice can you share with other acne sufferers?

Play around with your diet. Whether you do a formal elimination diet (which you can read about online) or just cut things out without recording and rotating. You'll be really, REALLY surprised how much a super "clean" diet affects your health. The government will tell you that you need to eat dairy for your bones or you'll see everyone else eating bread and think it's just fine, but when you cut those things out and feel 5 times better, lose weight and look terrific, you'll realize that those things we were brought up to think of as "healthy" may not really be that good for you. (P.S. you can get your calcium in other ways. Asian cultures didn't eat dairy for centuries and they also didn't suffer from our Western diseases until they *added* dairy, wheat and lots of red meat to their diets.)

Danielle Stallings began her career as a stage actor. She currently teaches film history in Los Angeles. She is an award-winning filmmaker whose recent achievements include the 35mm films "Haunted Planet" and "Up Under the Roof", both adapted from classic literary pieces.

KEVIN RAMAN

When did you discover that you had acne prone skin?
It started in High school. The pimples seemed mainly related to food, particularly if I ate chocolate.

Did you see a dermatologist? If so, was medication prescribed? What were the results?

I didn't see a dermatologist at the time. I *did* see a dermatologist when I was an adult, with good results.

What dietary changes, if any, did you make in an effort to control your acne?

I had to stay away from chocolate and greasy foods.

Did you make any non-dietary changes to your lifestyle in order to control acne?

Washing my face at night helped and avoiding touching my face with my hands

What do you think causes the kind of acne you have? Are there any specific triggers you can point to?

In my adult life the main trigger is stress. If I get stressed or don't get enough rest I breakout.

Do you take medication or use any types of drugs to treat your acne now? If so, which ones?

The one thing that works best for me now is a prescription medicine called Evoclin. It comes in a foam and really works best for me in stopping breakouts and speeding up the healing time when I do get a breakout.

Do you use any kinds of food or supplements to control your acne? If so, what do you use?

I drink aloe vera juice (which I got from you).

Do you exercise? If so, what do you do, and do you think it has any effect on your skin?

I haven't been exercising that much recently but salsa dancing helps cause I am constantly perspiring and I feeling like it opens the pores and gets a lot of the toxins out.

When your skin has been its best what were you doing?

Now is the best my skin has looked in years (I think it is just controlling stress and making better choices about the foods you take into your body.) I am eating mostly organic food now and although I am far from a health nut I have minimized a lot of the junk in my diet.

What advice can you share with other acne sufferers?

The pimples I had resulted in very dark scarring marks that would then last several months to years before they would fade. It made me very self conscious as a result. I rarely looked people straight in the eyes. I was always trying to hide my blemishes on my forehead with hats sunglasses and sweatbands. In some ways I let it affect my social life and my self confidence... I would say this: try to get the right treatment, of course, but while dealing with it, don't stop living your life.

Kevin Raman is a television editor and segment producer working in New York City. He's edited commercials, music videos and network television, including the David Letterman Show. He's a world traveler and avid Salsa dancer.

Acknowledgments

Many thanks to Leonard Chang, Vera Johnson, Nicole Sconiers, Dan Charnas, Rena Hecht, Heather Hamilton, Lisa Ruiz, Ann Marsh, Richard, Jo-Ann and Ri-Ann Pully, Mauren Regan, Monique Matthews, Lisa M. Pitt, Danielle Stallings, Kevin Raman, Reyna Grande, Jessica Garrison, Lisa Richardson, Sonia Nazario, and Lara Bazelon, for your input and encouragement on the Vibrating Youth series. Thanks to Adenrele Ojo for the book's author photos.

Toni Ann Johnson is a beauty and anti-aging specialist and author of *VIBRATING YOUTH,* available on Amazon.com.